HANDBOOK of

RADIOGRAPHIC POSITIONING and TECHNIQUES

NINTH EDITION

John P. Lampignano, MEd, RT(R)(CT)
Leslie E. Kendrick, MS, RT(R)(CT)(MR)

ELSEVIER

ELSEVIER

3251 Riverport Lane
St. Louis, Missouri 63043

Notices

Knowledge and best practice in this field are constantly changing. As new research and experience
broaden our understanding, changes in research methods, professional practices, or medical
treatment may become necessary.

Practitioners and researchers must always rely on their own experience and knowledge in
evaluating and using any information, methods, compounds, or experiments described herein. In
using such information or methods they should be mindful of their own safety and the safety of
others, including parties for whom they have a professional responsibility.

With respect to any drug or pharmaceutical products identified, readers are advised to check the
most current information provided (i) on procedures featured or (ii) by the manufacturer of each
product to be administered, to verify the recommended dose or formula, the method and duration
of administration, and contraindications. It is the responsibility of practitioners, relying on their
own experience and knowledge of their patients, to make diagnoses, to determine dosages and the
best treatment for each individual patient, and to take all appropriate safety precautions.

To the fullest extent of the law, neither the Publisher nor the authors, contributors, or editors,
assume any liability for any injury and/or damage to persons or property as a matter of products
liability, negligence or otherwise, or from any use or operation of any methods, products,
instructions, or ideas contained in the material herein.

Previous edition copyrighted 2014 by Mosby, an imprint of Elsevier Inc.
Previous edition copyrighted 2010 by Mosby, Inc., an affiliate of Elsevier Inc.
Previous editions copyrighted 2002, 1999, 1995, 1994 by Kenneth L. Bontrager

International Standard Book Number: 978-0-323-48525-8

Executive Content Strategist: Sonya Seigafuse
Content Development Manager: Lisa P. Newton
Senior Content Development Specialist: Tina Kaemmerer
Publishing Services Manager: Julie Eddy
Senior Project Manager: Mary G. Stueck
Design Direction: Renée Duenow

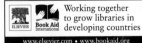

Printed in the United States of America

Last digit is the print number: 9   8   7   6   5   4   3   2   1

Preface

This pocket handbook was first developed by Kenneth Bontrager in 1994 as a response to the need felt by students and technologists for a more thorough but still practical pocket guide covering the applied aspects of radiographic positioning and techniques (exposure factors). Today, this compact and durable pocket-sized handbook includes a review of all the common imaging procedures, yet it is small enough to be easily carried in clinical situations. Sufficient space is included for writing personal notes and exposure factors that technologists find are optimal for specific equipment or in certain rooms or departments. Careful attention has been given to ensure the information on positioning in the Bontrager text is reflected accurately in the handbook.

Positioning descriptions and photographs are provided for each projection/position, along with CR locations, degrees of obliquity, specific CR angles, AEC cell locations, patient shielding, and suggested kV ranges for analog and digital systems. A quick review of this information before beginning a procedure can ensure the examination is being correctly performed, reducing the need for repeat exposures as a result of poor positioning or improper exposure factors.

Standard Radiographic Image and Evaluation Criteria

The ninth edition of this handbook includes a standard, well-positioned radiograph with each position described. Also added is a brief summary of quality factors to use an image evaluation matrix. Viewing this radiograph and comparing it with the list of evaluation criteria leads users through a critique of the image they are viewing for comparison to this standard.

Also included is an optional competency sign-off checksheet that can be signed by the clinical instructor for individual student competency records.

Acknowledgments

We would like to thank **Kelli Haynes, MSRS, RT(R),** who edited the 9th edition of the handbook. Kelli did an outstanding job updating the content in an extremely short time frame. This handbook is made possible through her expertise and attention to detail.

Sonya Seigafuse, Tina Kaemmerer, and Mary Stueck from Elsevier were instrumental in providing support, guidance, and the resources in the redesign and publishing of the pocket handbook. We are most indebted to our former students, fellow technologists, and those many educators throughout the United States and in the international imaging community who challenged and inspired us. We thank all of you and hope this pocket handbook continues to be a valuable aid in improving and maintaining that high level of radiographic imaging for which we all strive.

John and Leslie

Contents

Contents

v

Explanations for Use

This handbook is intended as a quick reference and review of radiographic positioning and procedures. It is not intended to replace the positioning techniques described in the Bontrager text. Rather, it is an ancillary tool that provides the technologist a quick review of the critical elements on positioning, CR location, kV ranges, and methods for reducing patient dose. These critical elements include:

Radiation protection: Certain radiation protection practices and shielding descriptions are included with each projection, and **it is the responsibility of the technologist to ensure that shielding** of radiosensitive tissues, collimation, and proper exposure factors are applied for each examination. Recommendations **for reducing patient dose are described in Appendix A.**

kV ranges: Suggested kV ranges for analog and digital systems are **stated** for each projection. These are recommendations based on best practices and validated by imaging experts. **These kV ranges may not apply to every department protocol or imaging systems employed.** The technologist should consult with his or her radiation safety officer or supervisor to determine appropriate kV ranges for their clinical setting.

Chapter title pages: The list of projections with page numbers is at the beginning of each chapter for ease in locating specific projections and also as a reference for marking the basic department routines for each examination. A small check ($\sqrt{}$) can be placed in the box by each projection that is part of the preferred departmental routine. Each projection is also followed by either an **(R)** or a **(S)** for a suggested departmental **routine** or **special.**

Standard Radiographic Image and Evaluation Criteria: Associated with each positioning page is a **radiograph** of that projection. These radiographs demonstrate the critical anatomy that must be visualized. A list of **evaluation criteria** is provided for the technologists to critique the images they have produced.

Also included is an optional **competency sign-off area** to be signed by the clinical instructor for individual student competency records.

Each positioning page has a format similar to this sample page.

1. Suggested location of patient ID information with analog imaging. For chest examinations, this represents the top right of the image receptor (IR).

2. Recommended AEC chamber(s) (darkened R and L upper cells indicated on this PA chest example). *Note:* Verify AEC chamber selection with department before employing.

3. Collimation field size with CR location in center.

4. IR size recommended for an average adult, placed portrait (lengthwise) or landscape (crosswise) in reference to the anatomy of interest. Grid or nongrid.

5. Patient position description.

6. CR location and CR angle.

7. Suggested SID range.

8. Suggested kV ranges. Analog and digital systems. (Pencil in kV range for your imaging systems.)

9. Exposure factors to be filled in (in pencil) as determined best for small (S), medium (M), or large (L) patients.

10. This additional space is provided for exposure factors for analog systems or for specific types of digital image receptors that require technique adjustments.

11. Corresponding page number in textbook for detailed information on the projection.

PA Chest

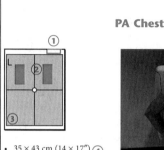

Fig. 1.2 P
below ve
female, 18

- 35 × 43 cm (14 × 17″) **(4)** portrait or landscape
- Grid

Position **(5)**
- Erect, chin raised, hands on hips with pa forward
- Center CR to the center of the lung field with accurate collimation on both top a
- Center thorax bilaterally to IR borders sides; ensure there is **no rotation** of tho

Central Ray: CR ⊥ to IR, centered to T7 **(6)** rtebra prominens (is also near level of in

SID: 72–120″ (183–307 cm) **(7)**

Collimation: Upper border to vertebra pro margins

Respiration: Expose at end of **second dee**

kV Range: **(8)** Analog and Digital Sy

	cm	kV	mA	Time	mAs
(9) S					
M	**(10)**				
L					

4   **(11)** Bontrager Textbook, 9th

Explanations for Use

vii

Chapter 1

Chest

Chest

1

Positioning Considerations and Radiation Protection

Collimation

Restricting the primary beam coverage is a very effective way to reduce patient exposure in chest radiography. This requires accurate and correct location of the central ray (CR).

Correct CR Location

Correct CR location to the midchest (T7) allows for accurate collimation and protection of the upper radiosensitive region of the neck area. It also prevents exposure to the dense abdominal area below the diaphragm, which produces scatter and secondary radiation to the radiosensitive reproductive organs.

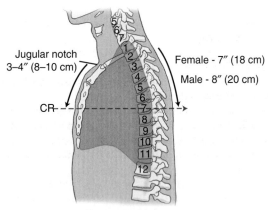

Jugular notch
3–4″ (8–10 cm)

Female - 7″ (18 cm)

Male - 8″ (20 cm)

CR

Fig. 1.1 Correct CR location.

T7 for the **PA chest** can be located posteriorly in reference to C7, the **vertebra prominens.** Level of T7 is 18–20 cm (7–8 inches) below the vertebra prominens.

The CR for the **AP chest** is 8–11 cm (3–4 inches) below the **jugular notch** and angled 3°–5° caudad (CR perpendicular to midsternum).

Shielding

Shielding of radiosensitive organs and tissues should be used for all procedures unless it obscures key anatomy. Shielding is not a substitute for close collimation.

Backscatter Protection

Shields placed between the patient and the wall bucky and wall can also be used to keep scatter and secondary radiation from these structures from reaching the patient's gonadal regions.

Digital Imaging Considerations

The following technical factors will reduce dose to the patient and improve image quality:

Collimation: Close collimation reduces dose to the patient and scatter radiation reaching the image receptor.

Accurate Centering: Most digital systems recommend that the anatomy be centered to the receptor.

Exposure Factors: Digital systems are known for wide exposure latitude, utilizing a broad range of exposure factors (kV and mAs). However, the ALARA principle must be followed, therefore, the highest kV and lowest mAs, consistent with optimal image quality, should be used.

Exposure Indicator (EI): Check the EI to verify that the optimal exposure factors were in the correct range to ensure optimal image quality and the least amount of radiation to the patient. Keep in mind that EI ranges are established by the manufacturers of the system and validated by your imaging department.

Grids: With certain digital systems, the grid may or may not be able to be removed from the receptor. In those cases, it is departmental protocol that determines whether a grid is left in place or removed.

PA: Chest

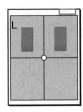

- 35 × 43 cm (14 × 17″) portrait or landscape
- Grid

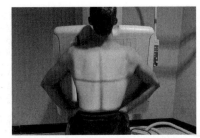

Fig. 1.2 PA chest (CR ≈20 cm [8″] below vertebra prominens) (average female, 18 cm [7″]).

Position
- Erect, chin raised, hands on hips with palms out, roll shoulders forward
- Center CR to the center of the lung fields on **all types** of patients with accurate collimation on both top and bottom
- Center thorax bilaterally to IR borders with equal margins on both sides; ensure there is **no rotation** of thorax

Central Ray: CR ⊥ to IR, centered to T7, or 7–8″ (18–20 cm) below vertebra prominens (is also near level of inferior angle of scapula)

SID: 72″ (183 cm)

Collimation: Upper border to vertebra prominens; sides to outer skin margins

Respiration: Expose at end of **second deep inspiration**

	cm	kV	mA	Time	mAs	SID	Exposure Indicator
kV Range:				Analog and Digital Systems: 110–125 kV			
S							
M							
L							

Bontrager Textbook, 9th ed, pp. 92–93.

Lateral: Chest

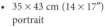

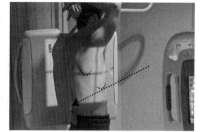

Fig. 1.3 Left lateral chest.

- 35 × 43 cm (14 × 17")
  portrait
- Grid

Position
- Erect, left side against IR (unless right lateral is indicated)
- Arms raised, crossed above head, chin up
- **True lateral**, no rotation or tilt. Midsagittal plane parallel to IR
  (Don't push hips in against the IR holder)
- Thorax centered to CR, and to IR anteriorly and posteriorly

Central Ray: CR ⊥ to IR, centered to midthorax at level of T7; generally IR and CR should be lowered ≈1" (2.5 cm) from PA on average patient

SID: 72" (183 cm)

Collimation: Upper border to level of vertebra prominens, sides to anterior and posterior skin margins

Respiration: Expose at end of **second full inspiration**

kV Range:			Analog and Digital Systems: 110–125 kV				
	cm	kV	mA	Time	mAs	SID	Exposure Indicator
S							
M							
L							

Lateral (Wheelchair or Stretcher): Chest

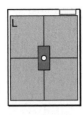

- 35 × 43 cm (14 × 17″) portrait
- Grid

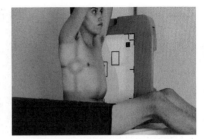

Fig. 1.4 Left lateral on stretcher.

Position
- Erect, on stretcher or in wheelchair
- Arms raised, crossed above head, or hold on to support bar
- Center thorax to CR, and to IR anteriorly and posteriorly
- No rotation or tilt, midsagittal plane parallel to IR, keep chin up

Central Ray: CR ⊥ to IR, centered to midthorax at level of T7

SID: 72″ (183 cm)

Collimation: Upper border to level of vertebra prominens, sides to anterior and posterior skin margins

Respiration: Expose at end of **second full inspiration**

kV Range:					Analog and Digital Systems: 110–125 kV	
	cm	kV	mA	Time	mAs	SID	Exposure Indicator
S							
M							
L							

Bontrager Textbook, 9th ed, p. 95.

PA (AP): Chest

Evaluation Criteria

Anatomy Demonstrated

- Both lungs from apices to costophrenic angles, and both lateral borders of ribs
- 10 ribs demonstrated above the diaphragm

Position

- Chin sufficiently elevated
- No rotation, SC joints and lateral rib margins equal distance from midline of spine

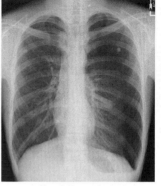

Fig. 1.5 PA chest.

Competency Check: _____
Technologist   Date

Chest

Exposure

- No motion, sharp outlines of diaphragm and lung markings visible
- Exposure sufficient to visualize faint outlines of midthoracic and upper thoracic vertebrae through heart and mediastinal structures

---

Lateral: Chest

Evaluation Criteria

Anatomy Demonstrated

- From apices to costophrenic angles, from sternum to posterior ribs

Position

- Chin and arms elevated to prevent superimposing apices
- No rotation, R and L posterior ribs superimposed except side away from IR projected slightly (1 cm) posteriorly because of divergent rays

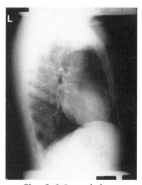

Fig. 1.6 Lateral chest.

Competency Check: _____
Technologist Date

Exposure

- No motion, sharp outlines of diaphragm and lung markings
- Sufficient exposure and contrast to visualize rib outlines and lung markings through heart shadow

7

Lateral Decubitus: Chest

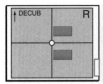

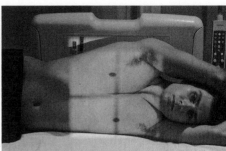

- 35 × 43 cm (14 × 17") portrait with respect to patient
- Grid

Position

Fig. 1.7 Left lateral decubitus chest (AP).

- Patient on side
  (R or L, see *Note*) with pad under patient
- Ensure that stretcher does not move (lock wheels)
- Raise both arms above head, chin up
- True AP, no rotation, patient centered to CR at level of T7

Central Ray: CR horizontal to T7, 3–4" (8–10 cm) below jugular notch

SID: 72" (183 cm) with wall bucky; 40–44" (102–113 cm) with erect table and bucky

Collimation: Collimate on four sides to area of lung fields (top border of light field to level of vertebra prominens)

Respiration: End of **second full inspiration**

Note: For possible fluid (pleural effusion), suspected side down; possible air (pneumothorax), suspected side up.

	cm	kV	mA	Time	mAs	SID	Exposure Indicator
S							
M							
L							

kV Range: Analog and Digital Systems: **110–125 kV**

Bontrager Textbook, 9th ed, p. 97.

AP Lordotic: Chest

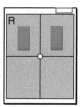

- 35 × 43 cm (14 × 17″) portrait
- Grid

Position
- Patient stands ≈1 ft (30 cm) away from IR, leans back against chest board
- Hands on hips, palms out, shoulders rolled forward
- Center midsternum and IR to CR, top of **IR** should be 7–8 cm (3″) above shoulders

Central Ray: CR ⊥ to IR, centered to midsternum (3–4 inches [9 cm] below jugular notch)

SID: 72″ (183 cm)

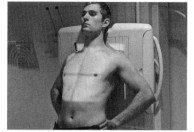

Fig. 1.8 AP lordotic (best demonstrates apices of lungs).

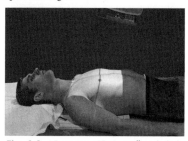

Fig. 1.9 AP supine, CR 15–20″ cephalad.

Collimation: Collimate on four sides to area of lung fields (top border of light field to level of vertebra prominens)

Respiration: End of **second full inspiration**

Note: If patient is too weak and unstable or is unable to assume the erect lordotic position, perform AP semiaxial projection with 15°–20° cephalad angle.

kV Range:			Analog and Digital Systems: 110–125 kV			
	cm	kV	mA	Time	mAs	SID	Exposure Indicator
S							
M							
L							

Chest

Lateral Decubitus: Chest

Evaluation Criteria

Anatomy Demonstrated

- Entire lung fields, including apices and costophrenic angles

Position

- No rotation, equal distance from lateral rib borders to spine

Exposure

- No motion; diaphragm, ribs, and lung markings appear sharp

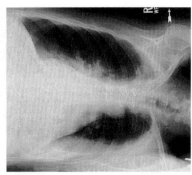

Fig. 1.10 Left lateral decubitus.

Competency Check: _____
Technologist   Date

- Faint visualization of vertebrae and ribs through heart shadow

---

AP Lordotic: Chest

Evaluation Criteria

Anatomy Demonstrated

- Entire lung fields; include clavicles, which should appear above apices

Position

- Clavicles appear nearly horizontal, superior to apices
- No rotation as evident by equal distance between medial ends of clavicles and lateral borders of ribs and midline of spine

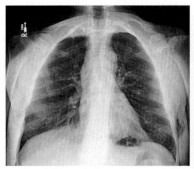

Fig. 1.11 AP lordotic chest.

Competency Check: _____
Technologist   Date

Exposure

- No motion; diaphragm, heart, and rib borders appear sharp
- Optimal contrast and density (brightness and contrast for digital images) to visualize vertebral outlines through mediastinal structures

Anterior Oblique (RAO and LAO): Chest

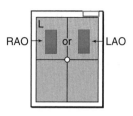

RAO → ← or → ← LAO

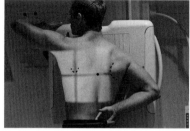

Fig. 1.12 45° RAO.

- 35 × 43 cm (14 × 17″) portrait
- Grid

Position
- Erect, rotated 45°, right anterior shoulder against IR for RAO and rotated 45° with left anterior shoulder against IR for LAO (Certain heart studies require LAO, 60° rotation from PA)
- Alternative posterior oblique positions can be performed. LPO best demonstrated left thorax and RPO the right thorax
- Arm away from IR up resting on head or on IR holder
- Arm nearest IR down on hip, keep chin raised
- Center thorax laterally to IR margins; vertically to CR at T7

Central Ray: CR ⊥ to IR, centered to level of T7 (7–8 inches [8–10 cm] below level of vertebra prominens)

SID: 72″ (183 cm)

Collimation: Collimate on four sides to area of lung fields (top border of light field to level of vertebra prominens)

Respiration: End of **second full inspiration**

---

kV Range:				Analog and Digital Systems: 110–125 kV		

	cm	kV	mA	Time	mAs	SID	Exposure Indicator
S							
M							
L							

Evaluation Criteria

Anatomy Demonstrated

- Included both lung fields from apices to costophrenic angles; RAO will elongate left thorax, and LAO will elongate right thorax

Position

- With 45° rotation, distance from outer rib margins to vertebral column on side farthest from IR should be approximately 2 times distance of side closest to IR

Exposure

- No motion; diaphragm and rib margins appear sharp
- Vascular markings throughout lungs and rib outlines visualized faintly through heart

Notes

- Anterior oblique positions best demonstrate the side farthest from IR. Posterior oblique positions best demonstrate the side closest to IR.
- Less rotation (15°–20°) may help better visualize areas of lungs for possible pulmonary disease.

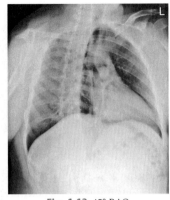

Fig. 1.13 45° RAO.

Competency Check: _____
Technologist   Date

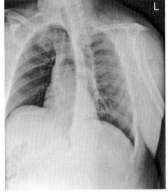

Fig. 1.14 45° LAO.

Competency Check: _____
Technologist   Date

AP and Lateral: Upper Airway
Trachea and Larynx

- 24 × 30 cm (10 × 12″) portrait
- Grid

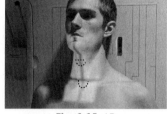

Fig. 1.15 AP.

Position
- Erect, seated or standing, center upper airway to CR
- Arms down, chin raised slightly
- Lateral: depress shoulders, and pull shoulders back
- Center of IR to level of CR

Central Ray: CR ⊥ to IR, centered to level of C6 or C7, midway between the laryngeal

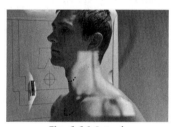

Fig. 1.16 Lateral.

prominence of the thyroid cartilage and the jugular notch

SID: 72″ (183 cm)

Collimation: Collimate to region of soft tissue neck

Respiration: Expose during slow, deep inspiration

	cm	kV	mA	Time	mAs	SID	Exposure Indicator
kV Range:			Analog and Digital systems: 75–85 kV				
S							
M							
L							

AP and Lateral: Upper Airway

Evaluation
Criteria
**Anatomy
Demonstrated
AP and Lateral**
- Larynx and
  trachea well
  visualized,
  filled with air

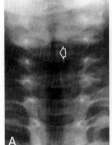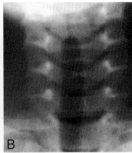

Fig. 1.17 AP upper airway.

Competency Check: _____
Technologist   Date

**Position
AP**
- No rotation,
  symmetric
  appearance of SC joints
- Mandible superimposes base of
  skull

Lateral
- To visualize neck region, include
  external auditory meatus at upper
  border of image.
- If distal larynx and trachea is of
  primary interest, center lower to
  include area from C3 to T5 (Fig.
  1.18).

**Exposure
AP**
- Optimal exposure visualizes
  air-filled trachea through C and
  T vertebrae

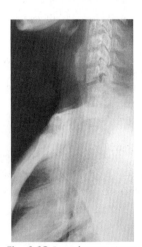

Fig. 1.18 Lateral upper airway.

Competency Check: _____
Technologist   Date

Lateral
- Optimal exposure includes air-
  filled larynx, and upper trachea
  not overexposed
- Cervical and thoracic vertebrae will appear underexposed

AP (Tabletop): Pediatric Chest

- 18 × 24 cm or 24 × 30 cm (8 × 10″ or 10 × 12″) landscape
- Nongrid; grid with digital systems when it cannot be removed

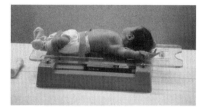

Fig. 1.19 Immobilization device.

Position

- Supine, arms and legs extended, tape and sandbags or other immobilization of arms and legs
- No rotation of thorax, gonadal shield over pelvic area
- IR and thorax centered to CR, with shoulders 5 cm (2″) below top of IR

Central Ray: CR ⊥ to IR, centered to midlung fields, mammillary (nipple) line

SID: Minimum 50–60″ (128–153 cm); x-ray tube raised as high as possible

Collimation: Closely collimate on four sides to outer chest margins

Respiration: Second full inspiration; if crying, time the exposure at full inhalation

Note: If parental assistance is necessary, have parent hold child's arms overhead tilting head back with one hand and holding down legs with other hand (provide lead apron and gloves).

	cm	kV	mA	Time	mAs	SID	Exposure Indicator
S							
M							
L							

kV Range: Analog and Digital Systems: 75–85 kV

Chest

1

Erect PA (With Pigg-O-Stat): Pediatric Chest

- 18 × 24 cm or 24 × 30 cm (8 × 10″ or 10 × 12″) landscape
- Nongrid or grid with systems when it cannot be removed

Position

- Patient on seat, legs through openings
- Adjust height of seat to place shoulders 2.5 cm (≈1″) below upper margin of IR
- Raise arms, and gently but firmly place side body clamps to hold raised arms and head in place
- Set upper border of lead shield with R and L markers 2.5–5 cm (1–2″) above level of iliac crest

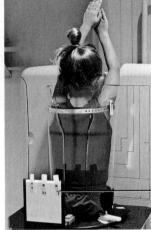

Markers and shield

Fig. 1.20 PA chest (Pigg-O-Stat, for 5-year-old) (DR).

Central Ray: CR ⊥ to IR, centered to midlung fields, mammillary (nipple) line

SID: Minimum of 72″ (183 cm)

Collimation: Collimate closely on four sides to outer chest margins

Respiration: Full inspiration; if crying, expose at full inhalation

kV Range:			Analog and Digital Systems: 75–85 kV			
	cm	kV	mA	Time	mAs	SID	Exposure Indicator
S							
M							
L							

Bontrager Textbook, 9th ed, p. 628.

Lateral (Tabletop): Pediatric Chest

- 18 × 24 cm or 24 × 30 cm (8 × 10″ or 10 × 12″) portrait
- Nongrid or grid with systems when it cannot be removed

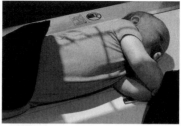

Fig. 1.21 Lateral chest (with tape and sandbags).

Chest

Position

- Lying on side (typically left lateral), arms up with head between arms
- Support arms with tape and sandbags; ensure a true lateral
- Flex legs; secure with tape and sandbags or with retention band across legs and hips; lead shield over pelvic region

Central Ray: CR ⊥ to IR, centered to midlung fields, level of mammillary (nipple) line

SID: Minimum of 50–60″ (128–153 cm); x-ray tube raised as high as possible

Collimation: Closely collimate on four sides to outer chest margins

Respiration: **Second full inspiration**; if crying, time exposure at full inhalation

Note: If parental assistance is necessary, have parent hold child's arms overhead, tilting head back with one hand and holding down legs with other hand (provide lead apron and gloves).

kV Range:					Analog and Digital Systems: 75–85 kV		
	cm	kV	mA	Time	mAs	SID	Exposure Indicator
S							
M							
L							

Erect Lateral (With Pigg-O-Stat): Pediatric Chest

- 18 × 24 cm or 24 × 30 cm (8 × 10″ or 10 × 12″) portrait
- Nongrid or grid with systems when it cannot be removed

Position

- With patient remaining in same position as for PA chest, change IR and rotate entire seat and body clamps 90° into a left lateral position; lead shield just above iliac crest
- Change lead marker to indicate left lateral

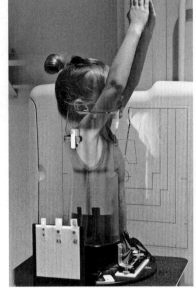

Fig. 1.22 Lateral chest (Pigg-O-Stat, for 5-year-old).

Central Ray: CR ⊥ to IR, centered to midlung fields, mammillary (nipple) line

SID: 72″ (183 cm)

Collimation: Closely collimate on four sides to outer chest margins

Respiration: Full inspiration; if crying, time exposure at full inhalation

| kV Range: | | | | Analog and Digital Systems: 75–85 kV | | | |

	cm	kV	mA	Time	mAs	SID	Exposure Indicator
S							
M							
L							

Bontrager Textbook, 9th ed, p. 630.

PA (AP): Pediatric Chest

Evaluation Criteria

Anatomy Demonstrated

- Entire lungs from apices to costophrenic angles

Position

- Chin elevated sufficiently
- No rotation, equal distance from lateral rib margins to spine
- Full inspiration, visualizes 9 (occasionally 10) posterior ribs above diaphragm

Exposure

- No motion, sharp outlines of rib margins and diaphragm
- Faint outline of ribs and vertebrae through heart and mediastinal structures

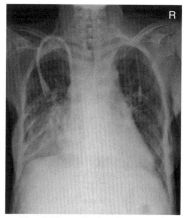

Fig. 1.23 AP (PA) pediatric chest (breathing and voluntary motion is evident, blurred diaphragm).

Competency Check: _____

Technologist   Date

Lateral: Pediatric Chest

Evaluation Criteria

Anatomy Demonstrated

- Entire lungs from apices to costo-phrenic angles and from sternum anteriorly to posterior ribs

Position

- Chin and arms elevated sufficiently
- No rotation, bilateral posterior ribs and costophrenic angles are superimposed

Exposure

- No motion; sharp outline of diaphragm, rib borders, and lung markings

Fig. 1.24 Lateral pediatric chest (DR).

Competency Check: _____

Technologist   Date

- Sufficient exposure to faintly visualize ribs and lung markings through heart shadow

19

Chapter 2

Upper Limb

Upper Limb

Forearm

Elbow

Pediatric Upper Limb

(R) Routine, (S) Special

Upper Limb

2

Technical Factors

The following technical factors are important for all upper limb procedures to maximize image sharpness.

- 40″ (102 cm) SID, minimum OID
- Small focal spot
- Nongrid or TT (tabletop), detail (analog) screens
- Digital imaging requires special attention to **accurate CR and part centering** and **close collimation.**
- Short exposure time
- Immobilization (when needed)
- **Multiple exposures per imaging plate:** Multiple images can be placed on the same IP. When doing so, careful collimation and lead masking must be used to prevent preexposure or fogging of other images. However, one exposure per imaging plate is recommended.
- **Grid use with digital systems:** Grids generally are not used with analog (film-screen) imaging for body parts measuring 10 cm or less. However, with certain digital systems, the grid may or may not be able to be removed from the receptor. In those cases, it is departmental protocol that determines whether a grid is left in place or removed. **Important:** If a grid is used, the anatomy must be centered to avoid grid cutoff.

Radiation Protection

Collimation
Close collimation is the most effective practice for preventing unnecessary radiation exposure to the patient.

Patient Shielding
Erect Patients: Patients seated at the end of the table should **always have a shield over radiosensitive organs** to prevent exposure from scatter radiation and from the divergent primary beam.
Recumbent Patients: A good practice to follow for upper limb examinations for patients on a stretcher or table is to always have shielding in place, especially the gonadal region.

PA: Fingers

Alternative Routine: Include entire hand on PA finger projection for possible secondary trauma to other parts of hand (see PA Hand).

- 18 × 24 cm (8 × 10″) portrait
- Nongrid
- Lead masking with multiple exposures on same IR

Position

- Patient seated at end of table, elbow flexed 90° (lead shield on patient's lap)
- Pronate hand, separate fingers.
- Center and align long axis of affected finger(s) to portion of IR being exposed

Central Ray: CR ⊥, centered to PIP joint

SID: 40″ (102 cm)

Collimation: On four sides to area of interest and distal aspect of metacarpal

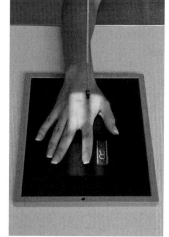

Fig. 2.1 PA—second digit.

kV Range:		Analog: 55 ± 5 kV		Digital Systems: 60 ± 5 kV		
	cm	kV	mA	Time	mAs	SID	Exposure Indicator
S							
M							
L							

PA Oblique: Fingers

- 18 × 24 cm (8 × 10″) portrait
- Nongrid
- Lead masking with multiple exposures on same IR

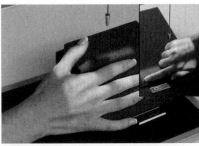

Fig. 2.2 PA oblique, second digit (parallel to IR). *Inset:* Minimized OID.

Position

- Patient seated, hand on table, elbow flexed 90° (lead shield on patient's lap)
- Align fingers to long axis of portion of IR being exposed
- Rotate hand 45° medially or laterally (dependent of digit examined), resting against 45° angle support block
- Separate fingers; ensure that affected finger(s) is (are) parallel to IR

Central Ray: CR ⊥, centered to PIP joint

SID: 40″ (102 cm)

Collimation: On four sides to area of affected finger(s) and distal aspect of metacarpal

kV Range: Analog: 55 ± 5 kV Digital Systems: 60 ± 5 kV

	cm	kV	mA	Time	mAs	SID	Exposure Indicator
S							
M							
L							

Bontrager Textbook, 9th ed, p. 143.

PA: Fingers

Evaluation Criteria

Anatomy Demonstrated
- Distal phalanx to distal metacarpal and associated joints

Position
- Long axis of digit parallel to IR with joints open
- No rotation of digit with symmetric appearance of shafts

Exposure
- Optimal density (brightness) and contrast
- Soft tissue margins and bony trabeculation clearly demonstrated; no motion

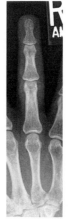

Fig. 2.3 PA finger.

Competency Check: _____
Technologist   Date

PA Oblique: Fingers

Evaluation Criteria

Anatomy Demonstrated
- Distal phalanx to distal metacarpal and associated joints

Position
- Interphalangeal and MCP joints open
- No superimposition of adjacent digits

Exposure
- Optimal density (brightness) and contrast
- Soft tissue margins and bony trabeculation clearly demonstrated; no motion

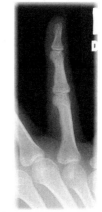

Fig. 2.4 PA oblique finger.

Competency Check: _____
Technologist   Date

Mediolateral and Lateromedial: Fingers

- 18 × 24 cm (8 × 10″) portrait
- Nongrid
- Lead masking with multiple exposures on same IR

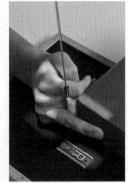

Fig. 2.5 Lateromedial fourth digit.

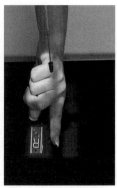

Fig. 2.6 Mediolateral second digit (digit parallel to IR).

Position
- Patient seated, hand on table (lead shield on patient's lap)
- Hand in lateral position, thumb side up for third to fifth digits, thumb side down for second digit
- Align finger to long axis of portion of IR being exposed

Central Ray: CR ⊥, centered to PIP joint

SID: 40″ (102 cm)

Collimation: On four sides to area of affected finger and distal aspect of metacarpal

kV Range:	Analog: 55 ± 5 kV			Digital Systems: 60 ± 5 kV		

	cm	kV	mA	Time	mAs	SID	Exposure Indicator
S							
M							
L							

Bontrager Textbook, 9th ed, p. 144.

AP: Thumb

- 18 × 24 cm (8 × 10″) portrait
- Nongrid
- Lead masking with multiple exposures on same IR

Position
- Patient standing or seated, hand rotated internally with palm out to bring the posterior surface of thumb in direct contact with IR
- Align thumb to long axis of portion of IR being exposed

Central Ray: CR ⊥, centered to first MCP joint

SID: 40″ (102 cm)

Collimation: Collimate closely to area of thumb (include entire first metacarpal extending to carpals)

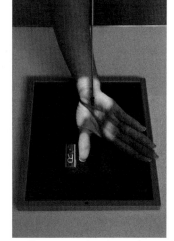

Fig. 2.7 AP thumb—CR to first MP joint.

Upper Limb

kV Range:	Analog: 55 ± 5 kV			Digital Systems: 60 ± 5 kV		
	cm	kV	mA	Time	mAs	SID	Exposure Indicator
S							
M							
L							

Lateral: Fingers

Evaluation Criteria

Anatomy Demonstrated

- Distal phalanx to distal metacarpal and associated joints

Position

- True lateral: joints are open and concave appearance of anterior surfaces of shaft of phalanges

Exposure

- Optimal density (brightness) and contrast
- Soft tissue margins and bony trabeculation clearly demonstrated; no motion

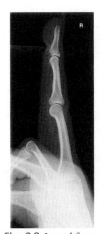

Fig. 2.8 Lateral finger.

AP: Thumb

Evaluation Criteria

Anatomy Demonstrated

- Distal phalanx to proximal metacarpal and trapezium

Position

- Long axis of thumb parallel to IR with joints open
- No rotation of thumb with symmetric appearance of shafts

Exposure

- Optimal density (brightness) and contrast
- Soft tissue margins and bony trabeculation clearly demonstrated; no motion

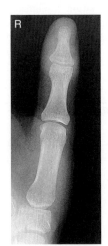

Fig. 2.9 AP thumb.

PA Oblique: Thumb

- 18 × 24 cm (8 × 10″) portrait
- Nongrid
- Lead masking with multiple exposures on same IR

Position

- Patient seated, hand on table, elbow flexed (shield on patient's R lap)
- Align thumb to long axis of portion of IR being exposed
- With hand pronated, abduct thumb slightly. This position tends to naturally rotate thumb into 45° oblique

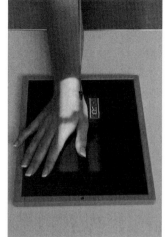

Fig. 2.10 PA oblique thumb, CR to first MCP joint.

Central Ray: CR ⊥, centered to first MCP joint
SID: 40″ (102 cm)
Collimation: Collimate closely to area of thumb (include entire first metacarpal extending to carpals)

	cm	kV	mA	Time	mAs	SID	Exposure Indicator
S							
M							
L							

kV Range: Analog: 55 ± 5 kV   Digital Systems: 60 ± 5 kV

2

Upper Limb

Lateral: Thumb

- 18 × 24 cm (8 × 10″) portrait
- Nongrid
- Lead masking with multiple exposures on same IR

Position
- Patient seated, hand on table, elbow flexed (shield on patient's lap)
- Align thumb to long axis of portion of IR being exposed
- With hand pronated and slightly arched, rotate hand medially until thumb is in true lateral position

Central Ray: CR ⊥, centered to first MCP joint
SID: 40″ (102 cm)
Collimation: Collimate closely to area of thumb (include entire first metacarpal extending to carpals)

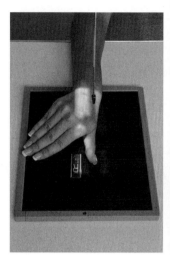

Fig. 2.11 Lateral thumb, CR to first MCP joint.

kV Range:		Analog: 55 ± 5 kV			Digital Systems: 60 ± 5 kV		
	cm	kV	mA	Time	mAs	SID	Exposure Indicator
S							
M							
L							

Bontrager Textbook, 9th ed, p. 147.

PA Oblique: Thumb

Evaluation Criteria
Anatomy Demonstrated
- Distal phalanx to proximal metacarpal and trapezium

Position
- Long axis of thumb parallel to IR with joints open

Exposure
- Optimal density (brightness) and contrast
- Soft tissue margins and bony trabeculation clearly demonstrated; no motion

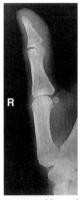

Fig. 2.12 PA oblique thumb.

Competency Check: _____

Technologist   Date

Lateral: Thumb

Evaluation Criteria
Anatomy Demonstrated
- Distal phalanx to proximal metacarpal and trapezium

Position
- True lateral position
- Interphalangeal and MCP joints open
- Anterior surfaces of first metacarpal and proximal phalanx equally concave shaped; posterior surfaces are relatively straight

Exposure
- Optimal density (brightness) and contrast
- Soft tissue margins and bony trabeculation clearly demonstrated; no motion

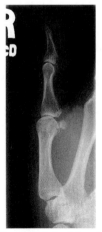

Fig. 2.13 Lateral thumb.

Competency Check: _____

Technologist   Date

31

AP Axial: Thumb
Modified Roberts Method

Note: This is a special projection to better demonstrate the **first carpometacarpal joint** region.

- 18 × 24 cm (8 × 10") portrait
- Nongrid
- Lead masking with multiple exposures on same IR

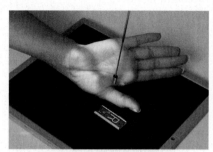

Fig. 2.14 AP axial thumb for first CMC joint (CR 15° proximally).

Position

- Patient seated or standing, hand rotated internally placing posterior surface of thumb directly on IR
- Align thumb to long axis of portion of IR being exposed.
- Extend

Central Ray: CR angled 15° proximally, centered to first CMC joint. The **Lewis modification** places the CR to the first MCP joint with a **10°–15°** proximal angle

SID: 40" (102 cm)

Collimation: Collimate closely to entire thumb, including the trapezium carpal bone

		kV Range:	Analog: 55 ± 5 kV		Digital Systems: 60 ± 5 kV		
	cm	kV	mA	Time	mAs	SID	Exposure Indicator
S							
M							
L							

Bontrager Textbook, 9th ed, p. 148.

PA: Hand

- 24 × 30 cm (10 × 12″) portrait
- Nongrid
- Lead masking with multiple exposures on same IR

Position
- Patient seated, hand on table, elbow flexed (shield on patient's lap)
- Align long axis of hand and wrist parallel to edge of IR
- Hand fully pronated, digits slightly separated

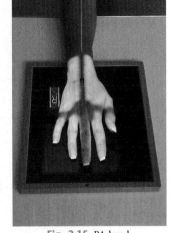

Fig. 2.15 PA hand.

Central Ray: CR ⊥, centered to third MCP joint

SID: 40″ (102 cm)

Collimation: Collimate on four sides to outer margins of hand and wrist. Include proximal and distal row of carpals

	kV Range:	Analog: 60–70 kV		Digital Systems: 60 ± 5 kV			
	cm	kV	mA	Time	mAs	SID	Exposure Indicator
S							
M							
L							

AP Axial: Thumb
Modified Roberts Method

Evaluation Criteria
Anatomy Demonstrated
- Distal phalanx to proximal metacarpal and trapezium
- Base of first metacarpal and trapezium well demonstrated

Position
- Long axis of thumb parallel to IR with joints open
- No rotation

Exposure
- Optimal density (brightness) and contrast
- Soft tissue margins and bony trabeculation clearly demonstrated; no motion

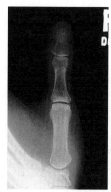

Fig. 2.16 AP axial thumb.

Competency Check: _____
Technologist   Date

PA: Hand

Evaluation Criteria
Anatomy Demonstrated
- Hand/wrist and 2.5 cm (1″) distal forearm

Position
- Interphalangeal and MCP joints open
- No rotation of hand with symmetric appearance of shafts of metacarpals and phalanges
- Digits slightly separated

Exposure
- Optimal density (brightness) and contrast
- Soft tissue margins and bony trabeculation clearly demonstrated; no motion

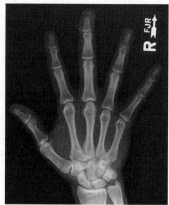

Fig. 2.17 PA hand.

Competency Check: _____
Technologist   Date

34

PA Oblique: Hand

- 24 × 30 cm (10 × 12″) portrait
- Nongrid
- Lead masking with multiple exposures on same IR

Position

- Patient seated, hand on table, elbow flexed (shield on patient's lap)
- Rotate entire hand and wrist laterally 45°, support with wedge or step block; align hand and wrist to IR
- Ensure that all digits are slightly separated and parallel to IR

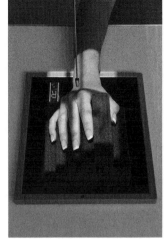

Fig. 2.18 PA oblique hand (digits parallel to IR).

Central Ray: CR ⊥, centered to third MCP joint
SID: 40″ (102 cm)
Collimation: Collimate on four sides to hand and wrist. Include proximal and distal row of carpals

	cm	kV	mA	Time	mAs	SID	Exposure Indicator
kV Range:		Analog: 60–70 kV			Digital Systems: 60 ± 5 kV		
S							
M							
L							

"Fan" Lateral and Lateral in Extension: Hand

- 18 × 24 cm (8 × 10″) portrait
- Nongrid
- Accessory—foam step support
- Lead masking with multiple exposures on same IR

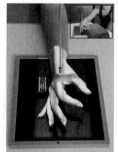

Fig. 2.19 "Fan" lateral hand (digits not superimposed).

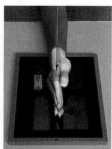

Fig. 2.20 Alternative: lateral in extension (for possible foreign body and metacarpal injury).

Position

- Patient seated, hand on table, elbow flexed (shield on patient's lap)
- Hand in lateral position, thumb side up, digits separated and spread into "fan" position and supported by radiolucent step block or similar type support (Ensure true lateral of metacarpals)

Central Ray: CR ⊥, centered to second MCP joint

SID: 40″ (102 cm)

Collimation: Collimate on four sides to hand and wrist. Include proximal and distal row of carpals

kV Range:	Analog: 60–70 kV			Digital Systems: 65 ± 5 kV		
	cm	kV	mA	Time	mAs	SID	Exposure Indicator
S							
M							
L							

PA Oblique: Hand

Evaluation Criteria

Anatomy Demonstrated

- Hand/wrist and 2.5 cm (1″) distal forearm

Position

- Long axis of digits/metacarpals parallel to IR with joints open
- No overlap of midshafts of third to fifth metacarpals

Exposure

- Optimal density (brightness) and contrast
- Soft tissue margins and bony trabeculation clearly demonstrated; no motion

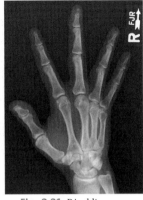

Fig. 2.21 PA oblique hand (digits parallel).

Competency Check: _____

Technologist   Date

"Fan" Lateral: Hand

Evaluation Criteria

Anatomy Demonstrated

- Hand/wrist and 2.5 cm (1″) distal forearm
- Interphalangeal and MCP joints open

Position

- Digits in true lateral position
- Phalanges and metacarpal surfaces symmetric
- Distal radius, ulna, and metacarpals superimposed

Exposure

- Optimal density (brightness) and contrast
- Soft tissue margins and bony trabeculation clearly demonstrated; no motion

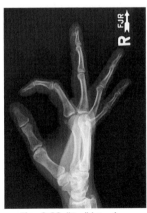

Fig. 2.22 "Fan" lateral hand.

Competency Check: _____

Technologist   Date

AP Oblique Bilateral: Hand
Norgaard Method and Ball-Catcher's Option

- 24 × 30 cm (10 × 12″) or 35 × 43 cm (14 × 17″) landscape
- Nongrid
- Accessories—two 45° foam sponges for support

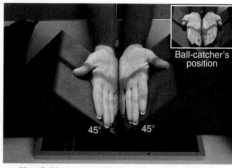

Ball-catcher's position

45°   45°

Fig. 2.23 AP 45° bilateral oblique. *Inset:* Ball-catcher's option.

Position

- Patient seated at end of table, both arms and hands extended with palms up and hands obliqued 45°, medial aspects touching
- Fingers fully extended supported by 45° support blocks

Ball-Catcher's Option:

- Fingers partially flexed, which visualizes metacarpals and MCP joints well but distorts interphalangeal joints

Central Ray: CR ⊥, centered to midway between fifth MCP joints
SID: 40″ (102 cm)
Collimation: Collimate to outer margins of hands and wrists. Include proximal and distal row of carpals

kV Range:		Analog: **60–70 kV**			Digital Systems: **60 ± 5 kV**	
	cm	kV	mA	Time	mAs	SID	Exposure Indicator
S							
M							
L							

Bontrager Textbook, 9th ed, p. 154.

AP Oblique Bilateral: Hand
Norgaard Method

Evaluation Criteria

Anatomy Demonstrated
- Both hands from carpals to distal phalanges
- Both hands positioned in 45° oblique

Position
- Midshafts of second to fifth metacarpals not overlapped
- MCP joints open

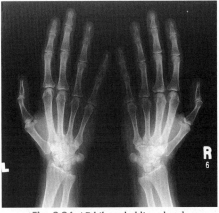

Fig. 2.24 AP bilateral oblique hand.

Competency Check: _____

Technologist   Date

Exposure
- Optimal density (brightness) and contrast
- Soft tissue margins and bony trabeculation with MCP joints clearly demonstrated to distal phalanges

PA: Wrist

- 18 × 24 cm (8 × 10″) portrait
- Nongrid
- Lead masking with multiple exposures on same IR

Position

- Patient seated, arm on table (shield on patient's lap)
- Align hand and wrist parallel to edge of IR
- Lower shoulder, rest arm on table to ensure no rotation of wrist
- Hand pronated, fingers flexed, and hand arched slightly to place wrist in direct contact with surface of IR

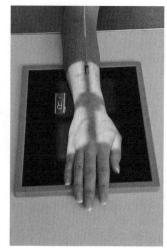

Fig. 2.25 PA wrist.

Central Ray: CR ⊥, centered to midcarpals

SID: 40″ (102 cm)

Collimation: Collimate to wrist on four sides. Include distal radius and ulna and the midmetacarpal area

kV Range:	Analog: 60–70 kV			Digital Systems: 60 ± 5 kV		
	cm	kV	mA	Time	mAs	SID	Exposure Indicator
S							
M							
L							

Bontrager Textbook, 9th ed, p. 155.

PA Oblique: Wrist

- 18 × 24 cm (8 × 10″) portrait
- Nongrid
- Lead masking with multiple exposures on same IR

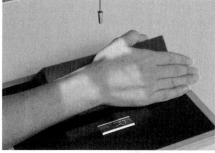

Fig. 2.26 45° PA oblique wrist (with support).

Position

- Patient seated, arm on table, elbow flexed (shield on patient's lap)
- Align hand and wrist parallel to edge of IR
- Rotate hand and wrist laterally into 45° oblique position
- Flex fingers to support hand in this position, or use 45° support sponge

Central Ray: CR ⊥, centered to midcarpals

SID: 40″ (102 cm)

Collimation: Collimate to wrist on four sides. Include distal radius and ulna and the midmetacarpal area

kV Range:		Analog: 60–70 kV		Digital Systems: 65 ± 5 kV		
	cm	kV	mA	Time	mAs	SID	Exposure Indicator
S							
M							
L							

PA: Wrist

Evaluation Criteria

Anatomy Demonstrated

- Midmetacarpals; carpals; distal radius, ulna, and associated joints

Position

- True PA is evidenced by symmetry of proximal metacarpals
- Separation of the distal radius and ulna

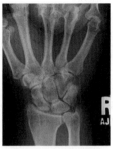

Fig. 2.27 PA wrist.

Competency Check: _____
                   Technologist   Date

Exposure

- Optimal density (brightness) and contrast
- Soft tissue margins and bony trabeculation of carpals clearly demonstrated; no motion

---

PA Oblique: Wrist

Evaluation Criteria

Anatomy Demonstrated

- Midmetacarpals; carpals; distal radius, ulna, and associated joints

Position

- Long axis of hand to forearm aligned to IR
- 45° oblique of wrist

Exposure

- Optimal density (brightness) and contrast
- Soft tissue margins and bony trabeculation of carpals clearly demonstrated; no motion

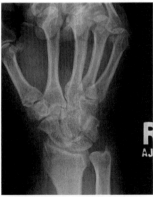

Fig. 2.28 PA oblique wrist.

Competency Check: _____
                   Technologist   Date

Lateral: Wrist

- 18 × 24 cm (8 × 10") portrait
- Nongrid
- Lead masking with multiple exposures on same IR

Position

- Patient seated, arm on table, elbow flexed, shoulder dropped to place humerus, forearm, and wrist on same horizontal plane (shield on patient's lap)
- Align hand and wrist parallel to edge of IR
- Place hand and wrist into a true lateral position, use support to maintain this position if needed

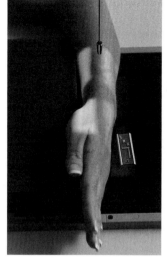

Fig. 2.29 Lateral wrist.

Central Ray: CR ⊥, centered to midcarpals

SID: 40" (102 cm)

Collimation: Collimate to wrist on four sides. Include distal radius and ulna and the midmetacarpal area

---

kV Range:	Analog: 60–70 kV			Digital Systems: 65 ± 5 kV		
	cm	kV	mA	Time	mAs	SID	Exposure Indicator
S							
M							
L							

2

Upper Limb

Evaluation Criteria
Anatomy Demonstrated
- Midmetacarpals; carpals; distal radius, ulna, and associated joints

Position
- True lateral of wrist
- Ulnar head superimposed distal radius

Exposure
- Optimal density (brightness) and contrast
- Soft tissue margins and bony trabeculation of carpals clearly demonstrated; no motion
- Demonstrate visible fat pads and stripes

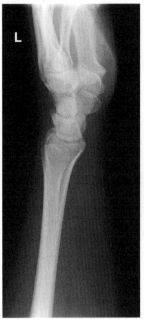

Fig. 2.30 Lateral wrist.

Competency Check: _____

Technologist   Date

PA and PA Axial With Ulnar Deviation: Scaphoid
10°–15° and Modified Stecher Method

Warning: The ulnar deviation projection should be attempted only with possible wrist trauma after a routine wrist series rules out gross fractures to wrist or distal forearm. PA axial projection recommended for obscure fractures. If patient can't ulnar deviate wrist, elevate hand on 20° angle sponge.

Note: See Chapter 1 in the 9th ed textbook for joint movement terminology.

- 18 × 24 cm (8 × 10″) portrait
- Nongrid
- Lead masking with multiple exposures on same IR

Position

- From PA wrist position, gently evert wrist toward ulnar side as far as patient can tolerate

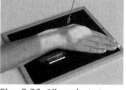

Fig. 2.31 Ulnar deviation, CR 10°–15° angle toward elbow. CR perpendicular to scaphoid.

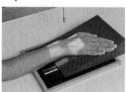

Fig. 2.32 Modified Stecher method. Elevate hand on 20° sponge, CR ⊥, to IR.

Central Ray: CR perpendicular to IR. Optional CR 10°–15° proximally toward elbow, centered to scaphoid (thumb side of carpal area); if hand placed on 20° sponge, CR ⊥ to IR

Note: A four-projection series with CR at 0°, 10°, 20°, and 30° may be required.

SID: 40″ (102 cm)

Collimation: Collimate on four sides to carpal region

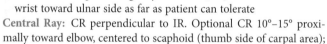

kV Range:	Analog: 60–70 kV			Digital Systems: 60 ± 5 kV			
	cm	kV	mA	Time	mAs	SID	Exposure Indicator
S							
M							
L							

Upper Limb

2

2

Upper Limb

Evaluation Criteria
Anatomy Demonstrated
- Scaphoid demonstrated clearly without foreshortening or overlap
- Soft tissue margins and bony trabeculation of scaphoid clearly demonstrated; no motion

Position
- Ulnar deviation evident
- Multiple CR angles may best visualize this area
- No rotation of wrist

Exposure
- Optimal density (brightness) and contrast
- Soft tissue margins and bony trabeculation of scaphoid clearly demonstrated; no motion

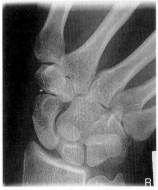

Fig. 2.33 Ulnar deviation with 10°–15° CR angle.

Competency Check: _____
Technologist   Date

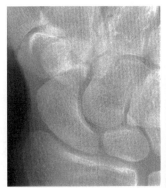

Fig. 2.34 Modified Stecher.

Competency Check: _____
Technologist   Date

PA With Radial Deviation: Wrist

Warning: This position should be attempted for possible wrist trauma only after a routine wrist series rules out gross fractures to wrist or distal forearm.

Note: See Chapter 1 in the 9th ed textbook, for explanation on wrist joint movement terminology.

- 18 × 24 cm (8 × 10″) portrait
- Nongrid
- Lead masking with multiple exposures on same IR

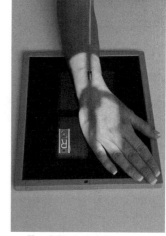

Fig. 2.35 Radial deviation, CR perpendicular. (Demonstrates ulnar side carpals.)

Position

- From PA wrist position, gently invert wrist toward radial side as far as patient can tolerate (shield across lap)

Central Ray: CR ⊥, to midcarpals

SID: 40″ (102 cm)

Collimation: Collimate closely to four sides of carpal region (≈7.5 cm or 3″ square)

kV Range:		Analog: **60–70 kV**			Digital Systems: **60 ± 5 kV**		

	cm	kV	mA	Time	mAs	SID	Exposure Indicator
S							
M							
L							

PA With Radial Deviation: Wrist

Evaluation Criteria

Anatomy Demonstrated
- Ulnar side carpals best visualized

Position
- Radial deviation evident
- No rotation of wrist

Exposure
- Soft tissue margins and bony trabeculation of ulnar aspect of carpal region clearly demonstrated; no motion
- Optimal density (brightness) and contrast

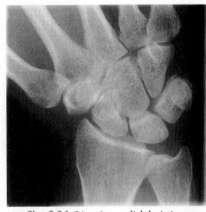

Fig. 2.36 PA wrist—radial deviation.

Competency Check: _____
Technologist   Date

Tangential Inferosuperior: Wrist (Carpal Canal)
Gaynor-Hart Method

Warning: This position is sometimes called the "tunnel view" and should be attempted for possible wrist trauma only after a routine wrist series rules out gross fractures to wrist or distal forearm.

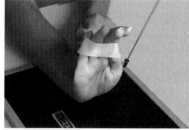

Fig. 2.37 Tangential (Gaynor-Hart method) projection (CR 25°–30° to long axis of hand).

- 18 × 24 cm (8 × 10″) portrait
- Nongrid
- Lead masking with multiple exposures on same IR

Position
- Patient seated, hand on table (shield on patient's lap)
- Hyperextend (dorsiflex) wrist as far as patient can tolerate with patient using other hand to hold fingers back
- Rotate hand and wrist slightly internally—toward radius (≈10°)
- Work quickly as this may be painful for patient

Central Ray: CR 25°–30° to long axis of the palmar surface of hand, centered to ≈1″ (2–3 cm) distal to base of third metacarpal

SID: 40″ (102 cm)

Collimation: Collimate to carpal region (≈7.5 cm or 3″ square)

| kV Range: | Analog: 60–70 kV | | | Digital Systems: 60 ± 5 kV | | |

	cm	kV	mA	Time	mAs	SID	Exposure Indicator
S							
M							
L							

Upper Limb

2

Tangential Inferosuperior: Wrist (Carpal Canal)
Gaynor-Hart Method

Evaluation Criteria

Anatomy Demonstrated
- Carpals demonstrated in arched arrangement

Position
- Pisiform and the hamular process separated (if not, wrist was not rotated 10° toward radius)
- Scaphoid/ trapezium in profile

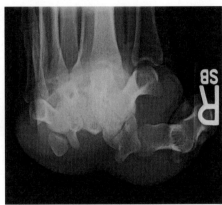

Fig. 2.38 Tangential (Gaynor-Hart).

Competency Check: _____
Technologist   Date

Exposure
- Optimal density (brightness) and contrast
- Soft tissue margins and bony trabeculation of carpal canal clearly demonstrated; no motion

AP: Forearm

- 35 × 43 cm (14 × 17″) portrait or 30 × 35 cm (11 × 14″) portrait for smaller patients
- Nongrid
- Lead masking with multiple exposures on same IR

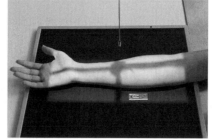

Fig. 2.39 AP forearm (to include both joints).

Position

- Patient seated at end of table with arm extended and hand supinated (shield on patient's lap)
- Ensure that both wrist and elbow joints are included (use as large an IR as required to include both wrist and elbow joints)
- Have patient lean laterally as needed for a true AP of forearm

Central Ray: CR ⊥, centered to midpoint of forearm

SID: 40″ (102 cm)

Collimation: Collimate on four sides. Include a minimum of 2.5 cm (1″) beyond both wrist and elbow joints

kV Range:		Analog: 65–75 kV		Digital Systems: 70 ± 5 kV			
	cm	kV	mA	Time	mAs	SID	Exposure Indicator
S							
M							
L							

Lateromedial: Forearm

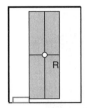

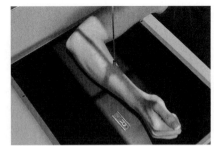

Fig. 2.40 Lateral forearm (to include both joints).

- 35 × 43 cm (14 × 17″) portrait or 30 × 35 cm (11 × 14″) portrait for smaller patients
- Nongrid
- Lead masking with multiple exposures on same IR

Position
- Patient seated at end of table (shield on patient's lap)
- Elbow should be flexed 90°
- Hand and wrist must be in a true lateral position (distal radius and ulna should be directly superimposed)
- Ensure that both wrist and elbow joints are included unless contraindicated

Central Ray: CR ⊥, centered to midpoint of forearm

SID: 40″ (102 cm)

Collimation: Collimate on four sides. Include a minimum of 2.5 cm (1″) beyond both wrist and elbow joints

kV Range:	Analog: 65–75 kV			Digital Systems: 70 ± 5 kV			
	cm	kV	mA	Time	mAs	SID	Exposure Indicator
S							
M							
L							

Bontrager Textbook, 9th ed, p. 165.

AP: Forearm

Evaluation Criteria
Anatomy Demonstrated
- Entire radius and ulna
- Entire elbow and proximal carpals

Position
- Slight superimposition of proximal radius/ulna
- Humeral epicondyles in profile

Exposure
- Optimal density (brightness) and contrast
- Soft tissue margins and bony trabeculation clearly demonstrated; no motion

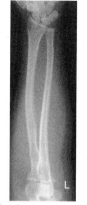

Fig. 2.41 AP forearm.

Competency Check: _____
Technologist   Date

2

Upper Limb

Lateromedial: Forearm

Evaluation Criteria
Anatomy Demonstrated
- Entire radius and ulna demonstrated
- Entire elbow and proximal carpals demonstrated

Position
- True lateral position
- Humeral epicondyles superimposed
- Head of ulna and distal radius are superimposed.

Exposure
- Optimal density (brightness) and contrast
- Soft tissue margins and bony trabeculation of carpal canal clearly demonstrated; no motion

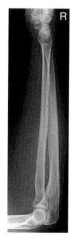

Fig. 2.42 Lateral forearm.

Competency Check: _____
Technologist   Date

53

AP: Elbow
Fully and Partially Extended

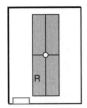

- 24 × 30 cm (10 × 12″) portrait
- Nongrid
- Lead masking with multiple exposures on same IR

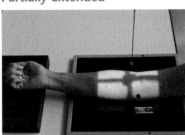

Fig. 2.43 AP, fully extended.

Position
- Elbow extended and hand supinated (shield on patient's lap)
- Lean laterally as needed for true AP (palpate epicondyles)
- If elbow cannot be fully extended, take two AP projections as shown (Figs. 2.44 and 2.45), with CR perpendicular to distal humerus on one and perpendicular to proximal forearm on another

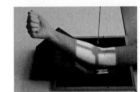

Fig. 2.44 CR, ⊥ to humerus.

Fig. 2.45 CR ⊥ to forearm.

Central Ray: CR ⊥, centered to midelbow joint

SID: 40″ (102 cm)

Collimation: Collimate on four sides to area of interest

kV Range:	Analog: 65–75 kV			Digital Systems: 70 ± 5 kV			
	cm	kV	mA	Time	mAs	SID	Exposure Indicator
S							
M							
L							

Bontrager Textbook, 9th ed, pp. 166 and 167.

AP: Elbow
Fully Extended

Evaluation Criteria

Anatomy Demonstrated
- Distal humerus
- Proximal radius and ulna

Position
- Slight superimposition of proximal radius/ulna
- Humeral epicondyles in profile

Exposure
- Optimal density (brightness) and contrast
- Soft tissue margins and bony trabeculation of elbow clearly demonstrated; no motion

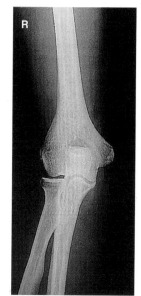

Fig. 2.46 AP elbow fully extended.

Competency Check: _____

Technologist   Date

AP: Elbow
Partially Flexed

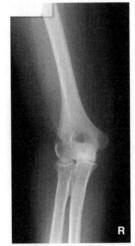

Fig. 2.47 Humerus parallel to IR.

Competency Check: _____
Technologist   Date

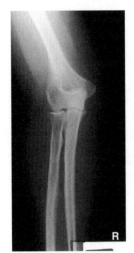

Fig. 2.48 Forearm parallel to IR.

Competency Check: _____
Technologist   Date

Evaluation Criteria
Anatomy Demonstrated

- Distal $\frac{1}{3}$ of humerus
- Proximal $\frac{1}{3}$ of forearm

Position

- Slight superimposition of proximal radius/ulna
- Humeral epicondyles in profile

Exposure

- Optimal density and contrast (brightness and contrast for digital images)
- Soft tissue and bony trabeculation clearly demonstrated; no motion

AP Oblique (Medial and Lateral): Elbow

Medial (internal) oblique best visualizes coronoid process. **Lateral (external) oblique** best visualizes radial head and neck (most common oblique projection).

- 24 × 30 cm (10 × 12″) portrait
- Nongrid

Position: Medial Oblique

- Elbow extended, hand pronated
- Palpate epicondyles to check for 45° internal rotation

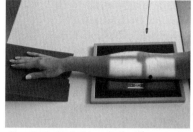

Fig. 2.49 Medial (internal) oblique (45°).

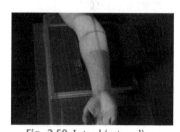

Fig. 2.50 Lateral (external) oblique (40°–45°).

Lateral Oblique: Similar position except supinate hand and rotate elbow 40°–45° externally. More difficult for patient; lean entire upper body laterally, as needed.

Central Ray: CR ⊥, centered to midelbow joint

SID: 40″ (102 cm)

Collimation: Collimate on four sides to area of interest

kV Range:		Analog: 65–75 kV			Digital Systems: 70 ± 5 kV	
	cm	kV	mA	Time	mAs	SID	Exposure Indicator
S							
M							
L							

AP Oblique (Medial): Elbow

Evaluation Criteria

Anatomy Demonstrated
- Proximal radius and ulna
- Medial epicondyle and trochlea

Position
- Coronoid process in profile
- Radial head/neck superimposed over ulna

Exposure
- Optimal density (brightness) and contrast
- Soft tissue margins and bony trabeculation clearly demonstrated

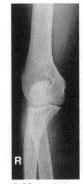

Fig. 2.51 Medial (internal) oblique elbow.

Competency Check: _____
Technologist   Date

AP Oblique (Lateral): Elbow

Evaluation Criteria

Anatomy Demonstrated
- Proximal radius and ulna
- Lateral epicondyle and capitulum

Position
- Radial head, neck, and tuberosity free of superimposition
- Humeral epicondyles and capitulum in profile

Exposure
- Optimal density (brightness) and contrast
- Soft tissue margins and bony trabeculation demonstrated; no motion

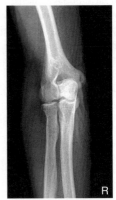

Fig. 2.52 Lateral (external) oblique elbow.

Competency Check: _____
Technologist   Date

Lateromedial: Elbow

- 24 × 30 cm (10 × 12″) portrait
- Nongrid
- Lead masking with multiple exposures on same IR

Position

- Elbow flexed 90°, shoulder dropped as needed to rest forearm and humerus flat on table and IR (shield on patient's lap)
- Center elbow to center of IR or to portion of IR being exposed, with forearm aligned parallel to edge of cassette
- Place hand and wrist in a true lateral position

Central Ray: CR ⊥, centered to midelbow joint

SID: 40″ (102 cm)

Collimation: Collimate on four sides. Include a minimum of ≈5 cm (2″) of forearm and humerus

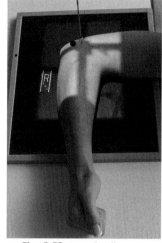

Fig. 2.53 Lateral—elbow flexed 90°.

2

Upper Limb

kV Range:		Analog: 60–70 kV		Digital Systems: 70 ± 5 kV			
	cm	kV	mA	Time	mAs	SID	Exposure Indicator
S							
M							
L							

Lateromedial: Elbow

Evaluation Criteria

Anatomy Demonstrated

- Proximal radius/ulna and distal humerus
- Region of joint fat pads

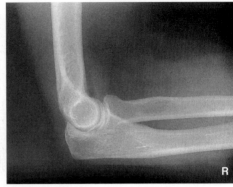

Fig. 2.54 Lateromedial elbow.

Competency Check: _____
Technologist   Date

Position

- Olecranon process/ trochlear notch in profile
- Radial head, neck, and tuberosity free of superimposition
- Humeral epicondyles superimposed
- Elbow flexed at 90°

Exposure

- Optimal density (brightness) and contrast
- Soft tissue margins and bony trabeculation clearly demonstrated

Axial Lateromedial and Mediolateral: Elbow (Trauma)
Coyle Method

Special views to demonstrate **radial head** and **coronoid process**
- 24 × 30 cm (10 × 12″) portrait
- Nongrid

Position and Central Ray

Radial Head:

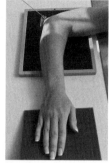

Fig. 2.55 For **radial head** and **neck**, elbow flexed **90°**.

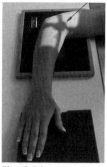

Fig. 2.56 For **coronoid process**, elbow flexed **80°**.

- Elbow flexed **90°** if possible, hand pronated
- Angle CR 45° toward shoulder, centered to radial head (CR to enter at midelbow joint)

Coronoid Process:
- Elbow flexed **only 80°**, with hand pronated
- Angle CR 45° away from shoulder, centered to coronoid process (CR to enter at midelbow joint)

SID: 40″ (102 cm)

Collimation: Collimate on four sides to area of interest

Upper Limb

	cm	kV	mA	Time	mAs	SID	Exposure Indicator
S							
M							
L							

kV Range: Analog: 65–75 kV*   Digital Systems: 70 ± 5 kV

*Increase exposure factors by 4–6 kV from lateral elbow because of angled CR.

Axial Lateromedial and Mediolateral: Elbow (Trauma)
Coyle Method

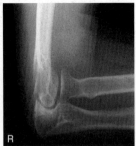

Fig. 2.57 Trauma axial lateral elbow (for radial head, neck, and capitulum).

Competency Check: _____
Technologist   Date

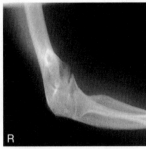

Fig. 2.58 Trauma axial lateral elbow (for coronoid process and trochlea).

Competency Check: _____
Technologist   Date

Evaluation Criteria

Anatomy Demonstrated and Position—Radial Head (CR 45° Toward Shoulder: Lateromedial Projection)

- Radial head, neck, and capitulum projected away from proximal ulna; elbow flexed **90°**

Anatomy Demonstrated and Position—Coronoid Process (CR 45° Away From Shoulder: Mediolateral Projection)

- Coronoid process and trochlea demonstrated
- Coronoid process in profile, elbow flexed **80°** (flexion of more than 80° will obscure coronoid process)

Exposure

- Optimal density (brightness) and contrast
- Soft tissue margins and bony trabeculation clearly demonstrated; no motion

AP: Upper Limb (Pediatric)

With possible trauma, handle limb very gently with minimal movement. Take a single exposure to rule out gross fractures before additional images are taken.

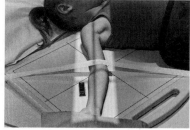

Fig. 2.59 AP—upper limb.

- IR size determined by patient age and size
- Nongrid

Position
- Supine position, arm abducted away from body, lead shield over pelvic area
- Include entire limb unless a specific joint or bone is indicated
- Immobilize with clear flexible-type retention band and sandbags, or with tape
- Use parental assistance only if necessary; provide lead gloves and apron

Central Ray: CR ⊥, centered to midlimb

SID: 40″ (102 cm)

Collimation: On four sides to area of interest

kV Range:		Analog: 55–65 kV			Digital Systems: 60–70 kV		
	cm	kV	mA	Time	mAs	SID	Exposure Indicator
S							
M							
L							

Lateral: Upper Limb (Pediatric)

- IR size determined by patient age and size
- Nongrid

Position
- Supine position with arm abducted away from body, lead shield over pelvic area

Fig. 2.60 Lateral—upper limb.

- Include entire limb unless a specific joint or bone is indicated
- Immobilize with clear flexible-type retention band and sandbags or with tape
- Flex elbow and rotate entire arm into a lateral position
- Use parental assistance only if necessary; provide lead gloves and apron

Central Ray: CR ⊥, centered to midlimb

SID: 40″ (102 cm)

Collimation: On four sides to area of interest

kV Range:	Analog: 55–65 kV				Digital Systems: 60–70 kV		
	cm	kV	mA	Time	mAs	SID	Exposure Indicator
S							
M							
L							

Bontrager Textbook, 9th ed, p. 631.

Chapter 3

Humerus and Shoulder Girdle

Important for humerus and shoulder projections: Do not attempt to rotate upper limb if fracture or dislocation is suspected without special orders by a physician.

(R) Routine, (S) Special

AP: Humerus

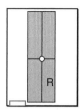

- 35 × 43 cm (14 × 17″) portrait or 30 × 35 cm (11 × 14″) portrait for small patients
- Grid >10 cm, IR only <10 cm

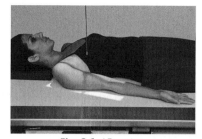

Fig. 3.1 AP supine.

Position
- Erect or supine with humerus aligned to long axis of IR (unless diagonal placement is needed to **include both elbow and shoulder joints**). Place shield over gonads
- Abduct arm slightly, supinate hand for true AP (epicondyles parallel to IR)

Central Ray: CR ⊥, to midhumerus
SID: 40″ (102 cm)

Collimation: Collimate on sides to soft tissue borders of humerus and shoulder

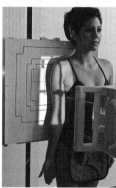

Fig. 3.2 AP erect.

3

Humerus and Shoulder Girdle

kV Range:		Analog: 70 ± 5 kV			Digital Systems: 80 ± 5 kV		
	cm	kV	mA	Time	mAs	SID	Exposure Indicator
S							
M							
L							

Rotational Lateral: Humerus

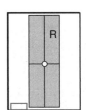

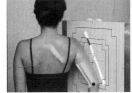

Fig. 3.3 Erect lateral (PA).

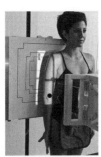

Fig. 3.4 Erect lateral (AP).

Warning: Do not attempt to rotate arm if fracture or dislocation is suspected (see following page).

- 35 × 43 cm (14 × 17″) or 30 × 35 cm portrait
- Grid >10 cm, IR only <10 cm

Position (May Be Taken Erect AP or PA, or Supine)

- **Erect (PA):** Elbow flexed 90°, patient rotated 15°–20° from PA or as needed to bring humerus and shoulder in contact with IR holder (epicondyles ⊥ to IR for true lateral)

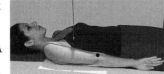

Fig. 3.5 Supine lateral.

- **Erect or supine AP:** Elbow slightly flexed, arm and wrist rotated for lateral position (palm back), epicondyles ⊥ to IR
- IR centered to **include both elbow and shoulder joints.** Shield radiosensitive tissues outside region of interest

Central Ray: CR ⊥, to midhumerus

SID: 40″ (102 cm)

Collimation: Collimate on sides to soft tissue borders of humerus and shoulder

kV Range:		Analog: 70 ± 5 kV			Digital Systems: 80 ± 5 kV		
	cm	kV	mA	Time	mAs	SID	Exposure Indicator
S							
M							
L							

Bontrager Textbook, 9th ed, p. 188.

Lateral: Humerus (Trauma)
Mid-to-Distal Humerus

For proximal humerus, see Transthoracic Lateral or Scapular Y.
- 30 × 35 cm (11 × 14″) landscape or 24 × 30 cm (10 × 12″) landscape
- Nongrid

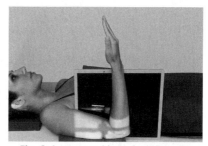

Fig. 3.6 Horizontal beam lateral cross-table, midhumerus and distal humerus.

Position
- Gently lift arm, and place support block under arm; rotate hand into lateral position, if possible, for true lateral elbow projection
- Place IR vertically between arm and thorax with top of IR at axilla (place shield between IR and patient)

Central Ray: CR horizontal and ⊥ to IR, centered to distal ⅓ of humerus

SID: 40″ (102 cm)

Collimation: Collimate on four sides. Include distal and midhumerus, elbow joint, and proximal forearm

kV Range:	Analog: 70 ± 5 kV			Digital Systems: 80 ± 5 kV		
	cm	kV	mA	Time	mAs	SID	Exposure Indicator
S							
M							
L							

AP and Lateral: Humerus

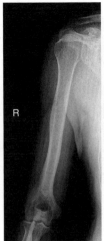

Fig. 3.7 AP humerus.

Competency Check: _____
           Technologist   Date

Fig. 3.8 Lateral erect humerus.

Competency Check: _____
         Technologist   Date

Evaluation Criteria

Anatomy Demonstrated

- AP and lateral view of the entire humerus, including elbow and glenohumeral joints

Position

AP

- No rotation, medial and lateral epicondyles seen in profile, greater tubercle in profile laterally
- Humeral head and glenoid cavity demonstrated

Lateral (PA)

- True lateral, epicondyles are directly superimposed

Exposure

- Optimal density (brightness) and contrast
- Sharp cortical margins and bony trabeculation clearly demonstrated, no motion

Transthoracic Lateral: Humerus (Trauma)

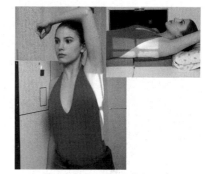

Fig. 3.9 Transthoracic lateral.

- 35 × 43 cm (14 × 17″) portrait
- Grid

Position
- Patient recumbent or erect
- Affected limb closest to IR
- Raise opposite arm over head

Central Ray: CR ⊥ to IR through midshaft of affected humerus
SID: 40″ (102 cm)
Collimation: To soft tissue margins—entire humerus
Respiration: Orthostatic (breathing) technique is preferred
If Orthostatic (Breathing) Lateral Technique Performed: Minimum of 3 seconds exposure time (between 4 and 5 seconds is desirable)

	cm	kV	mA	Time	mAs	SID	Exposure Indicator
kV Range:	Analog: 75 ± 5 kV			Digital Systems: 85 ± 5 kV			
S							
M							
L							

Transthoracic Lateral: Proximal Humerus

Evaluation Criteria

Anatomy Demonstrated

- Lateral view of the proximal half of humerus

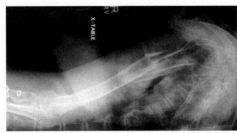

Fig. 3.10 Recumbent transthoracic lateral.

Position

- Proximal half of shaft of humerus should be clearly visualized
- Humeral head and glenoid cavity demonstrated

Exposure

- Optimal density (brightness) and contrast
- Overlying ribs and lung markings blurred (with breathing technique)

AP: Shoulder
External and Internal Rotation

Warning: Do not attempt if fracture or dislocation is suspected.

- 24 × 30 cm (10 × 12″) landscape (or lengthwise to show proximal aspect of humerus)
- Grid

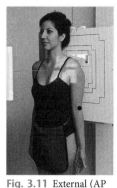

Fig. 3.11 External (AP "proximal" humerus).

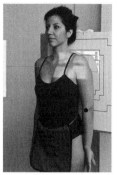

Fig. 3.12 Internal ("Proximal" lateral humerus).

Position

- Erect (seated or standing) or supine, arm slightly abducted
- Rotate thorax as needed to place posterior shoulder against IR
- Center of IR to scapulohumeral joint and CR

External Rotation: Rotate arm externally until hand is supinated and epicondyles are parallel to IR

Internal Rotation: Rotate arm internally until hand is pronated and epicondyles are perpendicular to IR.

Central Ray: CR⊥, directed to 1″ (2.5 cm) inferior to coracoid process

SID: 40″ (102 cm)

Collimation: Collimate closely on four sides

Respiration: Suspend during exposure

| kV Range: | Analog: 70–75 kV | | | Digital Systems: 80 ± 5 kV | | |

	cm	kV	mA	Time	mAs	SID	Exposure Indicator
S							
M							
L							

3

Humerus and Shoulder Girdle

AP: Shoulder
External and Internal Rotation

Evaluation Criteria

Anatomy Demonstrated

- Proximal humerus and lateral ⅔ of the clavicle (entire clavicle for crosswise IR) and upper scapula

Position

External Rotation

- Greater tubercle visualized in full profile laterally
- Lesser tubercle superimposed over humeral head

Internal Rotation (Lateral)

- Lesser tubercle visualized in full profile medially
- Greater tubercle superimposed over humeral head

Exposure

- Optimal density (brightness) and contrast
- Soft tissue detail and sharp bony trabeculation clearly demonstrated; no motion

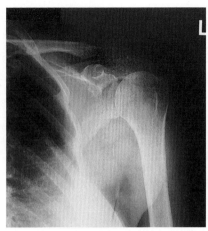

Fig. 3.13 External rotation—AP.

Competency Check: _____

Technologist   Date

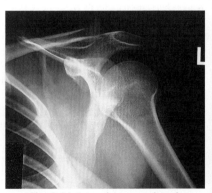

Fig. 3.14 Internal rotation—lateral.

Competency Check: _____

Technologist   Date

3

Humerus and Shoulder Girdle

Inferosuperior Axial: Shoulder
Lawrence Method

Warning: Do not attempt if fracture or dislocation is suspected.

- 18 × 24 cm (8 × 10″) landscape
- Grid; grid lines horizontal and CR to center line of grid
- Often performed nongrid for smaller shoulder

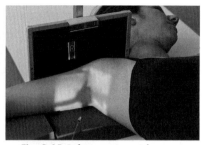

Fig. 3.15 Inferosuperior axial (Lawrence method).

Position

- Patient supine, to front edge of table or stretcher, with support under shoulder to center anatomy to IR, head turned away from IR
- Arm abducted 90° from body, if possible
- Rotate arm externally, with hand supinated

Note: An **alternative position** is exaggerated **external** rotation with the thumb is pointed down and posteriorly approximately 45°. Recommended in ruling out a Hills-Sachs defect

Central Ray: CR horizontal, directed 25°–30° medially to axilla, less angle if arm is not abducted 90° (place tube next to table or stretcher at same level as axilla)

SID: 40″ (102 cm)

Collimation: Collimate closely on four sides

Respiration: Suspend during exposure

| kV Range: | Analog: 70 ± 5 kV | | Digital Systems: 80 ± 5 kV | | | |

	cm	kV	mA	Time	mAs	SID	Exposure Indicator
S							
M							
L							

Inferosuperior Axial: Shoulder
Lawrence Method

Evaluation Criteria

Anatomy Demonstrated

- Lateral view of proximal humerus in relationship to the scapulohumeral cavity

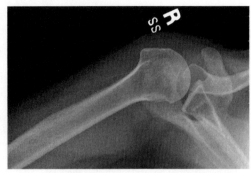

Fig. 3.16 Inferosuperior axial (Lawrence method).

Competency Check: _____

Technologist   Date

Position

- Spine of scapula is seen in profile inferior to the scapulohumeral joint
- Affected arm abducted about 90°

Exposure

- Optimal density (brightness) and contrast
- Soft tissue detail and sharp bony trabeculation clearly demonstrated; no motion

PA Transaxillary: Shoulder
Hobbs Modification

- 18 × 24 cm (8 × 10") portrait
- Grid

Position
- Patient recumbent or erect PA
- Affected arm raised superiorly and fully extended
- Head is turned away

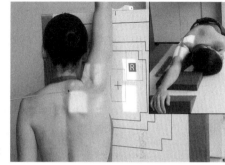

Fig. 3.17 PA transaxillary (Hobbs modification).

Central Ray: Perpendicular to the IR, centered to the glenohumeral joint

SID: 40" (102 cm)

Collimation: Collimate closely on four sides

Respiration: Suspend during exposure

kV Range:		Analog: 70 ± 5 kV		Digital Systems: 80 ± 5 kV			
	cm	kV	mA	Time	mAs	SID	Exposure Indicator
S							
M							
L							

Evaluation Criteria
Anatomy Demonstrated
- Lateral view of proximal humerus in relationship to scapulohumeral (glenohumeral) joint

Position
- Coracoid process of scapula is seen on end
- Affected arm elevated completely

Exposure
- Optimal density (brightness) and contrast
- Soft tissue and sharp bony trabeculation clearly demonstrated; no motion

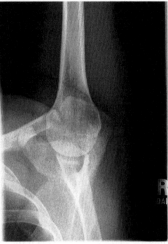

Fig. 3.18 PA transaxillary (Hobbs modification).

Competency Check: _____

               Technologist   Date

3

Humerus and Shoulder Girdle

Inferosuperior Axial: Shoulder
Clements Modification

- 18 × 24 cm (8 × 10″) portrait
- Nongrid (can use grid if CR is perpendicular to it)

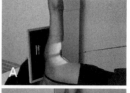

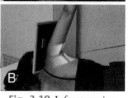

Fig. 3.19 Inferosuperior axial (Clements modification).

Position
- Lateral recumbent position; lying on unaffected side
- Affected arm up
- Abduct arm 90° from body, if possible

Central Ray: Direct horizontal CR perpendicular to the IR (Angle the tube 5°–15° toward the axilla if the patient cannot abduct the arm 90°)

SID: 40″ (102 cm)

Collimation: Collimate closely on four sides

Respiration: Suspend during exposure

3

Humerus and Shoulder Girdle

kV Range:	Analog: 70 ± 5 kV			Digital Systems: 80 ± 5 kV		
	cm	kV	mA	Time	mAs	SID	Exposure Indicator
S							
M							
L							

Inferosuperior Axial: Shoulder
Clements Modification

Evaluation Criteria

Anatomy Demonstrated
- Lateral view of proximal humerus in relationship to the scapulohumeral joint

Position
- Arm is abducted 90° from the body

Exposure
- Optimal density (brightness) and contrast
- Soft tissue and sharp bony trabeculation clearly demonstrated; no motion

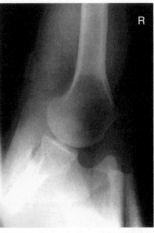

Fig. 3.20 Inferosuperior axial (Clements modification). (From Frank ED, Long BW, Smith BJ: *Merrill's atlas of radiographic positioning and procedures,* ed 11, St Louis, 2007, Mosby.)

Competency Check: _____
                    Technologist   Date

AP Oblique—Glenoid Cavity: Shoulder
Grashey Method

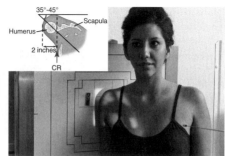

Fig. 3.21 AP oblique—Grashey method.

A special projection for visualizing glenoid cavity in profile with open joint space

- 18 × 24 cm (8 × 10″) landscape
- Grid

Position

- Erect or supine (erect preferred)
- Oblique 35°–45° toward side of interest (body of scapula should be parallel with IR), hand and arm in neutral rotation
- Center midscapulohumeral joint and IR to CR (5 cm [2″] inferior and medial from the superolateral border of shoulder)

Central Ray: CR ⊥, to scapulohumeral joint

SID: 40″ (102 cm)

Collimation: Collimate so upper and lateral borders of the field are to the soft tissue margins

Respiration: Suspend during exposure

kV Range: Analog: 75 ± 5 kV Digital Systems: 80 ± 5 kV

	cm	kV	mA	Time	mAs	SID	Exposure Indicator
S							
M							
L							

Humerus and Shoulder Girdle

3

AP Oblique: Shoulder
Grashey Method

Evaluation Criteria
Anatomy Demonstrated
- View of head of humerus in relationship to glenoid cavity

Position
- Open scapulohumeral joint space
- Anterior and posterior rims of glenoid cavity are superimposed.

Exposure
- Optimal density (brightness) and contrast
- Soft tissue margins and sharp bony trabeculation clearly demonstrated; no motion

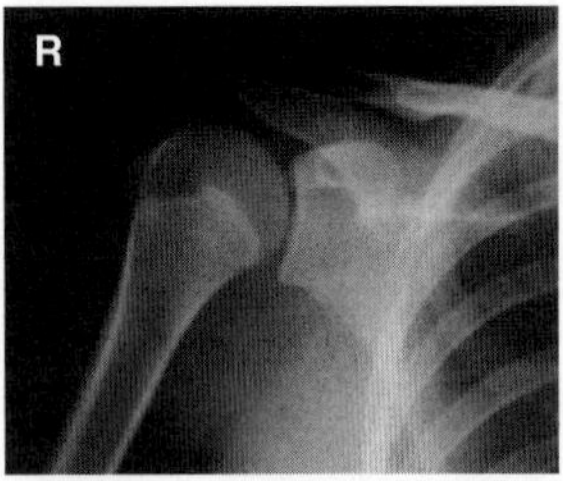

Fig. 3.22 AP oblique—Grashey method.

Competency Check: _____
Technologist   Date

Tangential—Intertubercular (Bicipital) Sulcus: Shoulder

Fisk Modification

- 18 × 24 cm (8 × 10″) landscape
- Nongrid

Position

- Supine or erect. Palpate anterior humeral head to locate groove

Supine: Abduct arm slightly, supinate hand

- Center IR and groove to CR.
- CR 10°–15° posterior from horizontal position of x-ray tube, centered to groove, IR vertical against top of shoulder, perpendicular to CR

Alternative Erect: Patient standing, leaning over the end of the table to place humerus 10°–15° from vertical, CR vertical, ⊥ to IR

SID: 40″ (102 cm)

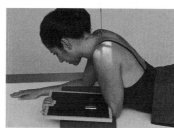

Fig. 3.23 Supine inferosuperior tangential projection (CR 15°–20° from horizontal).

Fig. 3.24 Erect superoinferior tangential (humerus 15°–20° from vertical, CR, ⊥ to IR).

Collimation: Collimate closely on four sides to area of anterior humeral head

Respiration: Suspend during exposure

	cm	kV	mA	Time	mAs	SID	Exposure Indicator
kV Range:		Analog: 70 ± 5 kV			Digital Systems: 75 ± 5 kV		
S							
M							
L							

Tangential—Intertubercular (Bicipital) Sulcus: Shoulder
Fisk Modification

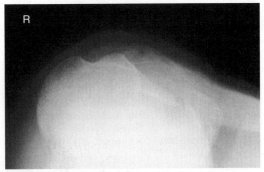

Fig. 3.25 Erect tangential projection (intertubercular groove).

Competency Check: _____

Technologist   Date

Evaluation Criteria
Anatomy Demonstrated
- Humeral tubercles and intertubercular groove seen in profile

Position
- Intertubercular groove and tubercles in profile
- No superimposition of acromion process

Exposure
- Optimal density (brightness) and contrast
- Sharp borders and sharp bony trabeculation clearly demonstrating intertubercular sulcus seen through soft tissue; no motion

PA Oblique: Shoulder (Trauma)
Scapular Y Lateral and Neer Method

- 24 × 30 cm (10 × 12″) portrait
- Grid

Position
- Erect or recumbent (erect preferred)
- Patient PA then rotate affected shoulder into a 45°–60° posterior oblique as for a lateral scapula (body of scapula perpendicular to IR)
- Unaffected arm up in front of patient, affected arm down **(don't move with possible fracture or dislocation)**
- Center scapulohumeral joint and CR

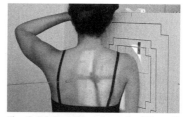

Fig. 3.26 PA oblique (scapular Y lateral) with CR ⊥.

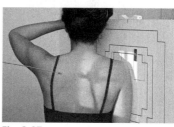

Fig. 3.27 Tangential (Neer method) with CR 10°–15° caudad.

Central Ray: CR ⊥ to scapulo-humeral joint

Neer Method: Angle CR 10°–15° caudad to better demonstrate the acromiohumeral space (supraspinatus outlet), CR to superior margin of humeral head

SID: 40″ (102 cm)

Collimation: Collimate on four sides to area of interest

Respiration: Suspend during exposure

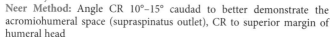

kV Range:		Analog: 75 ± 5 kV		Digital Systems: 80 ± 5 kV			
	cm	kV	mA	Time	mAs	SID	Exposure Indicator
S							
M							
L							

Humerus and Shoulder Girdle

3

PA Oblique: Shoulder (Trauma)
Scapular Y Lateral and Neer Method

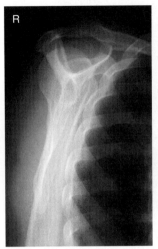

Fig. 3.28 PA oblique (scapular Y lateral) with no dislocation.

Competency Check: _____
Technologist   Date

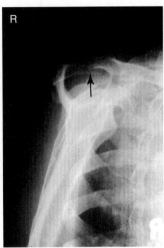

Fig. 3.29 Tangential projection (Neer method).

Competency Check: _____
Technologist   Date

Evaluation Criteria

Anatomy Demonstrated

- **Scapular Y:** True lateral view of the scapula, proximal humerus
- **Neer method:** Supraspinatus outlet region is open

Position

- **Scapular Y:** Thin body of the scapula seen on end without rib superimposition. Upper limb is not elevated or moved with possible fracture or dislocation
- **Neer method:** Thin body of the scapula seen on end; humeral head below supraspinatus outlet *(arrow)*

Exposure

- Optimal density (brightness) and contrast
- Bony margins clearly demonstrated; no motion

AP—Neutral Rotation: Shoulder (Trauma)

- 24 × 30 cm (10 × 12″) landscape (or portrait to show more of humerus if injury includes proximal half of humerus)
- Grid

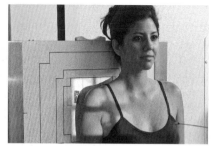

Fig. 3.30 AP—neutral rotation.

Note: Evaluation of AP shoulder-neutral position is similar to external/internal rotation, but neither the greater tubercle nor the lesser tubercle is in profile (if limb can be moved)

Position

- Erect (seated or standing) or supine, arm slightly abducted
- Rotate thorax slightly as needed to place posterior shoulder against IR
- Arm in neutral position (generally with palm inward—no acute trauma present)

Central Ray: CR ⊥, to ¾″ (2 cm) inferior to coracoid process
SID: 40″ (102 cm)
Collimation: Collimate on four sides to area of interest
Respiration: Suspend during exposure

kV Range:	Analog: 70–75 kV			Digital Systems: 80 ± 5 kV		
	cm	kV	mA	Time	mAs	SID	Exposure Indicator
S							
M							
L							

Transthoracic Lateral: Shoulder (Trauma)
Lawrence Method

- 24 × 30 cm (10 × 12″) portrait
- Grid
- Orthostatic (breathing) technique is preferred if patient can cooperate

Position

- Erect or supine, affected arm against IR, arm at side in neutral position
- Raise unaffected arm above head
- Elevate unaffected shoulder, **or** angle CR 10°–15° cephalad to prevent superimposition of unaffected shoulder
- True lateral, or slight anterior rotation of unaffected shoulder
- Center grid IR to CR

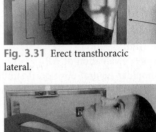

Fig. 3.31 Erect transthoracic lateral.

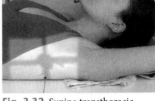

Fig. 3.32 Supine transthoracic lateral.

Central Ray: CR⊥, through thorax to surgical neck

SID: 40″ (102 cm)

Collimation: Collimate on four sides to area of interest

Respiration: Expose on full inspiration; orthostatic (breathing) technique preferred

kV Range:	Analog: 75 ± 5 kV			Digital Systems: 85 ± 5 kV		

	cm	kV	mA	Time	mAs	SID	Exposure Indicator
S							
M							
L							

Bontrager Textbook, 9th ed, p. 200.

Transthoracic Lateral: Shoulder (Trauma)
Lawrence Method

Evaluation Criteria

Anatomy Demonstrated

- Lateral view of proximal humerus and glenohumeral joint

Position

- Shaft of the proximal humerus should be clearly visualized
- Humeral head and the glenoid cavity visualized

Exposure

- Optimal density (brightness) and contrast
- Ribs and lungs should be blurred due to breathing technique, but bony outlines of the humerus should be sharp indicating no motion

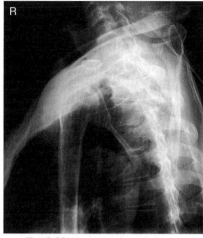

Fig. 3.33 Erect transthoracic lateral.

Competency Check: _____

Technologist   Date

Humerus and Shoulder Girdle

AP Apical Oblique Axial: Shoulder (Trauma)
Garth Method

A good projection for acute shoulder trauma, demonstrating shoulder dislocations, glenoid fractures, and Hill-Sachs lesions
- 24 × 30 cm (10 × 12″) portrait
- Grid

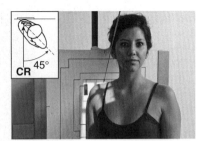

Fig. 3.34 Erect apical oblique (45° posterior oblique, CR 45° caudad).

Position
- Erect preferred (recumbent, if necessary)
- Rotate thorax 45° with affected shoulder against IR
- Flex affected elbow and place hand on opposite shoulder
- Center IR to exiting CR

Central Ray: CR 45° caudad, to medial aspect of scapulohumeral joint
SID: 40″ (102 cm)
Collimation: Collimate on four sides to area of interest
Respiration: Suspend during exposure

	cm	kV	mA	Time	mAs	SID	Exposure Indicator
S							
M							
L							

kV Range: Analog: 75 ± 5 kV   Digital Systems: 80 ± 5 kV

Bontrager Textbook, 9th ed, p. 203.

AP Apical Oblique Axial: Shoulder (Trauma)
Garth Method

Evaluation Criteria

Anatomy Demonstrated

- Humeral head, glenoid cavity, and neck and head of scapula free of superimposition

Position

- Acromion and AC joint projected superior to humeral head

Exposure

- Optimal density (brightness) and contrast
- Soft tissue detail and sharp bony trabeculation clearly demonstrated; no motion

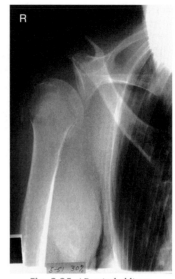

Fig. 3.35 AP apical oblique.

Competency Check: _____
 Technologist   Date

Humerus and Shoulder Girdle

Apical AP Axial: Shoulder

Demonstrates narrowing of acromiohumeral space and possible spurring of the anteroinferior aspect of acromion.

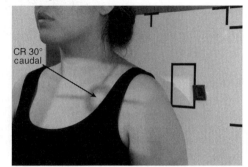

- 18 × 24 cm (8 × 10″) or 24 × 30 cm (10 × 12″) landscape
- Grid

Fig. 3.36 Erect apical AP axial (CR 30° caudad).

Position

- Erect preferred
- Position patient with no rotation
- Affected hand in neutral position

Central Ray: Angle CR 30° caudad entering ½″ (1.25 cm) above **coracoid process**

SID: 40″ (102 cm)

Collimation: Collimate to soft tissue margins of shoulder

Respiration: Expose upon suspended respiration

kV Range:		Analog: 75 ± 5 kV			Digital Systems: 80 ± 5 kV		
	cm	kV	mA	Time	mAs	SID	Exposure Indicator
S							
M							
L							

Bontrager Textbook, 9th ed, p. 197.

Apical AP Axial: Shoulder

Evaluation Criteria

Anatomy Demonstrated

- The anteroinferior aspect of the acromion process and acromiohumeral joint space is open
- Proximal humerus is projected in neutral rotation position

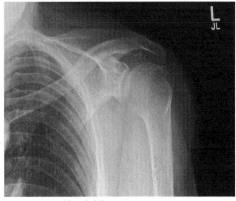

Fig. 3.37 Apical AP axial.

Competency Check: _____

Technologist   Date

Position:

- Acromiohumeral space is more open as compared to routine AP shoulder projection
- Anteroinferior aspect of acromion is demonstrated

Exposure

- Optimal density (brightness) and contrast
- Soft tissue detail and sharp bony trabeculation clearly demonstrated; no motion

Humerus and Shoulder Girdle

AP and AP Axial: Clavicle

- 24 × 30 cm (10 × 12″) landscape
- Grid

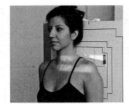

Fig. 3.38 AP, 0°.

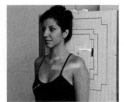

Fig. 3.39 AP axial, 15° to 30° cephalad.

Position

- Erect or recumbent
- Center clavicle and IR to CR (midway between jugular notch medially and AC joint laterally)

Central Ray: CR to midclavicle

AP: CR ⊥, to midclavicle

AP Axial: 15°–30° cephalad* (thin shoulders require 5°–15° more angle than thick shoulders)

Note: Departmental routines may include AP 0°, or axial AP, or both

SID: 40″ (102 cm)

Collimation: Collimate to area of clavicle (Ensure that both AC and sternoclavicular joints are included)

Respiration: Expose upon full inspiration

*AP lordotic position can be performed rather than angling CR for AP axial.

	kV Range:	Analog: 70 ± 5 kV		Digital Systems: 80 ± 5 kV		
	cm	kV	mA	Time	mAs	SID	Exposure Indicator
S							
M							
L							

Bontrager Textbook, 9th ed, p. 204.

AP and AP Axial: Clavicle

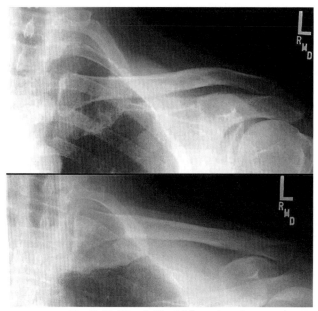

Fig. 3.40 AP and AP axial (lower image).

Competency Check: _____
Technologist   Date

Evaluation Criteria

Anatomy Demonstrated

- **AP 0°:** Entire clavicle including both AC and SC joints
- **AP axial:** The entire clavicle including both AC and SC joints above the scapula and ribs

Position

- **AP 0°:** Entire clavicle from AC to SC joint
- **AP axial:** Only medial portion of clavicle will be superimposed by first and second ribs

Exposure

- Optimal density (brightness) and contrast
- Soft tissue detail and sharp bony trabeculation clearly demonstrated; no motion

AP: Scapula

- 24 × 30 cm (10 × 12″) portrait
- Grid

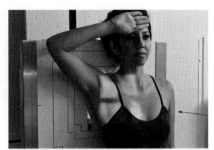

Fig. 3.41 AP scapula erect.

Position

- Erect or supine (erect preferred with pain in scapula area)
- Gently abduct arm 90°, if possible; supinate hand (abduction results in less superimposition of scapula by ribs)
- Center IR and entire scapula to CR

Central Ray: CR ⊥, to midscapula (2″ or ≈5 cm inferior to coracoid process and 2″ [5 cm] medial from lateral border of patient)

SID: 40″ (102 cm)

Collimation: Collimate on four sides of scapula borders.

Respiration: Breathing technique preferred can be employed or suspend respiration during exposure.

kV Range:	Analog: 75 ± 5 kV			Digital Systems: 80 ± 5 kV			
	cm	kV	mA	Time	mAs	SID	Exposure Indicator
S							
M							
L							

Bontrager Textbook, 9th ed, p. 207.

Lateral (Erect and Recumbent): Scapula

- 24 × 30 cm (10 × 12″) portrait

Position

- Erect or recumbent (erect preferred)

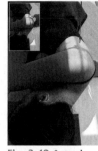

Fig. 3.42 Lateral (palpate scapular borders).

- Palpate borders of scapula and rotate thorax until body of scapula is perpendicular to IR (will vary from 45°–60° rotation)
- If area of interest is body of scapula, with patient's arm up, have patient reach across and grasp opposite shoulder

Central Ray: CR ⊥, to midvertebral border of scapula
SID: 40″ (102 cm)
Collimation: To scapular region
Respiration: Suspend during exposure

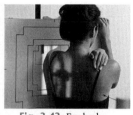

Fig. 3.43 For body of scapula.

Fig. 3.44 Superior scapula (acromion or coracoid process), place arm down, flex elbow, palm out.

kV Range:		Analog: 75 ± 5 kV			Digital Systems: 80 ± 5 kV		
	cm	kV	mA	Time	mAs	SID	Exposure Indicator
S							
M							
L							

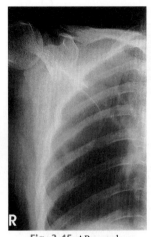

Fig. 3.45 AP scapula.

Competency Check: _____

Technologist   Date

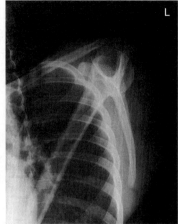

Fig. 3.46 Lateral scapula.

Competency Check: _____

Technologist   Date

Evaluation Criteria

Anatomy Demonstrated

- **AP:** Entire scapula
- **Lateral:** Entire scapula in a lateral position

Position

- **AP:** Lateral border of scapula free of superimposition
- **Lateral:** Humerus not superimposing over region of interest; ribs free of superimposition by body of scapula

Exposure

- Optimal density (brightness) and contrast
- Sharp bony borders and trabeculation clearly demonstrated; no motion

AP (Bilateral): Acromioclavicular (AC) Joints
Pearson Method, With and Without Weights

Warning: Rule out fracture before taking "with weight" projection.
- 35 × 43 cm (14 × 17″) or (2) 18 × 24 cm (8 × 10″) for broad shoulders, landscape
- Grid or nongrid (depending on size of shoulder)
- Use markers "with weights" and "without weights"

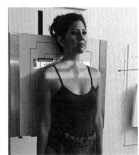

18 cm (8″)   24 cm (10″)   24 cm (10″)   (broad-shouldered patient)

Position
- Erect, standing if possible, or may be seated on chair
- Arms at sides, one exposure for bilateral without weights, and a second exposure with 8–10 lb minimum (5–8 lb for smaller patient) weights tied to wrists, shoulders and arms relaxed, center IR to CR

Fig. 3.47 Bilateral with weights.

Central Ray: CR ⊥, to midpoint between AC joints, 1″ (2.5 cm) above jugular notch

SID: 40″ (102 cm); 72″ (183 cm) recommended for bilateral studies with a single IR

Collimation: Long, narrow horizontal exposure field

Respiration: Suspend during exposure

Alternative AP Axial Projection (Alexander Method): A 15° cephalic angle centered at the level of the affected AC joint to rule out subluxation or dislocation of AC joint

	cm	kV	mA	Time	mAs	SID	Exposure Indicator
kV Range:	Analog: 65 ± 5 kV (70–75 kV with grid)			Digital Systems: 80 ± 5 kV (grid recommended for larger shoulders)			
S							
M							
L							

AP (Bilateral): AC Joint
Pearson Method, With and Without Weights

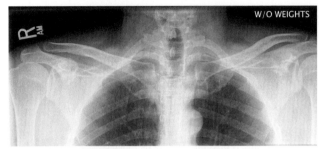

Fig. 3.48 AP acromioclavicular joints without weights.

Competency Check: _____
Technologist   Date

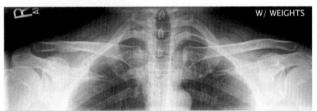

Fig. 3.49 AP acromioclavicular joints with weights.

Competency Check: _____
Technologist   Date

Evaluation Criteria
Anatomy Demonstrated
- Both R and L AC joints and SC joints included

Position
- No rotation, symmetric SC joints

Exposure
- Optimal density (brightness) and contrast; no motion
- Bony margins and sharp bony trabeculation clearly demonstrated

Chapter 4

Lower Limb

- Technical considerations and radiation protection 103

4

Lower Limb

(R) Routine, (S) Special

4

Lower Limb

Technical Considerations

The principal exposure factors for radiography of the lower limbs include the following:

- Low-to-medium kV (50–75); 70–80 digital systems
- Short exposure time
- Small focal spot
- Adequate mAs for sufficient density (brightness)
- Grids: for anatomy measuring >10 cm in thickness

Digital Imaging Considerations

- **Four-sided collimation:** Collimate to the area of interest with a minimum of two collimation parallel borders clearly demonstrated on the image. Four-sided collimation is always preferred.
- **Accurate centering:** It is important that the body part and the central ray be centered to the IR.
- **Grid use with cassette-less systems:** Anatomy thickness and kV range are deciding factors for whether a grid is to be used. With cassette-less systems it may be impractical and difficult to remove the grid. Therefore the grid is commonly left in place even for smaller body parts measuring 10 cm or less. If the grid is left in place, it is important to ensure that the CR is centered to the grid for all projections.

Radiation Protection
Collimation and Shielding

A general rule for protective shielding states that it should be used whenever radiation-sensitive areas lie within or near the primary beam. Red bone marrow and gonadal tissues are two of the key radiation-sensitive regions. However, a good practice to follow, in addition to **close collimation** to the area of interest, is to use **shielding** on youth and patients of childbearing age for **all** lower limb procedures. All radiosensitive tissues should be protected unless it involves area of interest. This provides assurance to the patient that he or she is being protected from unnecessary exposure.

Multiple Exposures per Imaging Plate

Placing multiple images on the same IP is not recommended. However, if doing so, careful collimation and lead masking must be used to prevent pre-exposure of other images.

AP: Toes

Alternative Routine: May include entire foot on AP toe projection for possible secondary trauma to other parts of foot (see AP foot).

- 18 × 24 cm (8 × 10")
  landscape
- Nongrid
- Lead masking with
  multiple exposures on
  same IR

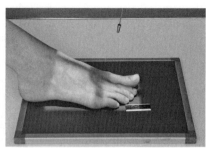

Fig. 4.1 AP second digit, CR 10°–15° toward calcaneus.

Position

- Supine or seated on table with knee flexed, plantar surface of foot resting on IR
- Align long axis of affected toe(s) to portion of IR being exposed

Central Ray:

- CR angled 10°–15° to calcaneus (⊥ to long axis of digits)
- CR centered to MTP joint(s) of interest

SID: 40" (102 cm)

Collimation: Collimate on four sides to area of interest to include soft tissue margins.

	cm	kV	mA	Time	mAs	SID	Exposure Indicator
kV Range:		Analog: 50–55 kV			Digital Systems: 60 ± 5 kV		
S							
M							
L							

AP Oblique: Toes

- 18 × 24 cm (8 × 10″) landscape
- Nongrid
- Lead masking with multiple exposures on same IR

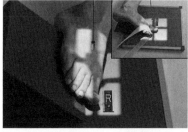

Fig. 4.2 Medial oblique rotation (first digit).

Position

- Supine or seated on table, foot resting on IR
- Align long axis of affected toe(s) to portion of IR being exposed
- Oblique foot 30°–45° medially for first to third digits, and laterally for fourth and fifth digits. Place support under foot as shown

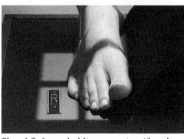

Fig. 4.3 Lateral oblique rotation (fourth digit).

Central Ray: CR ⊥, centered to MTP joint(s) of interest
SID: 40″ (102 cm)
Collimation: Collimate on four sides to area of interest to include soft tissues.

	cm	kV	mA	Time	mAs	SID	Exposure Indicator
S							
M							
L							

kV Range: Analog: 50–55 kV   Digital Systems: 60 ± 5 kV

4

Lower Limb

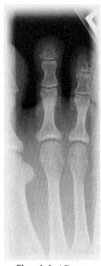

Fig. 4.4 AP toe.

Competency
Check: _____
       Technologist Date

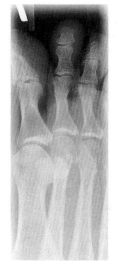

Fig. 4.5 Medial oblique toe.

Competency
Check: _____
       Technologist Date

Evaluation Criteria

Anatomy Demonstrated

- **AP and AP Oblique:** Entire digit and minimum of ½ of affected metatarsal

Position

- **AP:** No overlap of surrounding digits and metatarsals; no rotation, equal concavity on both sides of shafts of phalanges and metatarsals
- **AP Oblique:** Increased concavity on one side of phalangeal shaft

Exposure

- Optimal density (brightness) and contrast; no motion
- Sharp cortical margins and bony trabeculae clearly demonstrated

Lateral: Toes

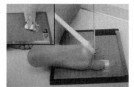

Fig. 4.6 Lateromedial (first digit).

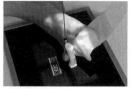

Fig. 4.7 Mediolateral (fourth digit).

- 18 × 24 cm (8 × 10") landscape
- Nongrid
- Lead masking with multiple exposures on same IR

Position
- Seated or recumbent on tabletop
- Carefully use tape and/or radiolucent gauze to isolate unaffected digits as shown:
  - First to third digits—lateromedial projection (first digit down)
  - Fourth to fifth digits—mediolateral projection (first digit up)

Central Ray: CR ⊥, to IP joint for first digit, and to PIP joint for second to fifth digits

SID: 40″ (102 cm)

Collimation: Collimate closely to digit of interest to include soft tissues

kV Range:	Analog: 50–55 kV			Digital Systems: 60 ± 5 kV			
	cm	kV	mA	Time	mAs	SID	Exposure Indicator
S							
M							
L							

4

Lower Limb

Tangential: Toes—Sesamoids

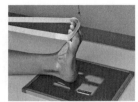

- 18 × 24 cm (8 × 10″) landscape
- Nongrid
- Lead masking with multiple exposures on same IR

Fig. 4.8 Patient prone.

Fig. 4.9 Alternative supine position.

Position

- Patient prone with foot and great toe carefully dorsiflexed so that the plantar surface forms a 15°–20° angle from vertical, if possible (adjust CR angle, as needed)

Alternative Supine Position: May be a more tolerable position for patient to maintain if in great pain. Long strip of gauze is needed for the patient to hold the toes as shown

Central Ray: CR ⊥, or angled, as needed, depending on amount of dorsiflexion of foot, centered to head of first metatarsal

SID: 40″ (102 cm)

Collimation: Collimate closely to area of interest; include distal first, second, and third metatarsals for possible sesamoids

kV Range:	Analog: 50–55 kV			Digital Systems: 60 ± 5 kV		
	cm	kV	mA	Time	mAs	SID	Exposure Indicator
S							
M							
L							

Bontrager Textbook, 9th ed, p. 231.

Evaluation Criteria
Anatomy Demonstrated
- Entire digit, including proximal phalanx

Position
- No superimposition of adjoining digits
- Proximal phalanx visualized through superimposed structures

Exposure
- Contrast and density (brightness) sufficient to visualize soft tissue and bony portions; no motion

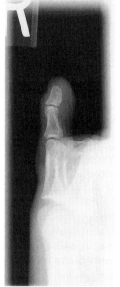

Fig. 4.10 Lateromedial second digit.

Competency
Check: _____
       Technologist   Date

4

Lower Limb

Tangential: Sesamoids

Evaluation Criteria
Anatomy Demonstrated
- Sesamoid bones in profile

Position
- No superimposition of sesamoids and first to third distal metatarsals in profile

Exposure
- Optimal density (brightness) and contrast; no motion
- Soft tissue, trabeculae, and sharp cortical margins clearly demonstrated

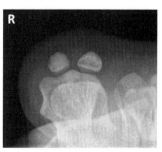

Fig. 4.11 Tangential sesamoids.

Competency
Check: _____
       Technologist   Date

109

Dorsoplantar AP: Foot

- 24 × 30 cm (10 × 12″) portrait
- Nongrid
- Lead masking with multiple exposures on same IR

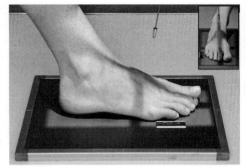

Fig. 4.12 AP foot, CR 10° posteriorly.

Position

- Supine or seated with plantar surface flat on IR, aligned lengthwise to portion of IR being exposed
- Extend (plantar flex) foot by sliding foot and IR distally while keeping plantar surface flat on IR (Support with sandbags to keep foot and IR from sliding farther)

Central Ray: CR ⊥, to metatarsals, which is about 10° posteriorly (toward heel), centered to base of third metatarsal

SID: 40″ (102 cm)

Collimation: Four sides to margins of foot

	cm	kV	mA	Time	mAs	SID	Exposure Indicator
S							
M							
L							

kV Range: Analog: 60 ± 5 kV   Digital Systems: 65 ± 5 kV

Bontrager Textbook, 9th ed, p. 232.

4

Lower Limb

AP Medial Oblique: Foot

- 24 × 30 cm (10 × 12″) portrait
- Nongrid
- Lead masking with multiple exposures on same IR

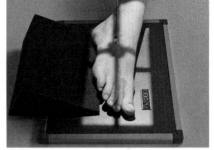

Fig. 4.13 30°–40° medial oblique.

Position

- Supine or seated with foot centered lengthwise to portion of IR being exposed
- Oblique foot 30°–40° medially, support with 45° radiolucent angle block and sandbags to prevent slippage
- **Note 1:** A higher arch requires nearer 45° oblique and a low arch "flat foot" nearer 30°
- **Note 2:** A 30° lateral oblique projection will demonstrate the space between first and second metatarsals and between first and second cuneiforms

Central Ray: CR ⊥, centered to base of third metatarsal

SID: 40″ (102 cm)

Collimation: Four sides to skin margins of foot and distal ankle

kV Range:	Analog: 60 ± 5 kV			Digital Systems: 65 ± 5 kV			
	cm	kV	mA	Time	mAs	SID	Exposure Indicator
S							
M							
L							

AP and AP Medial Oblique: Foot

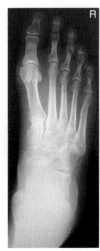

Fig. 4.14 AP foot.

Competency
Check: _____
Technologist   Date

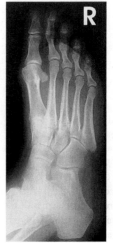

Fig. 4.15 Medial oblique foot.

Competency
Check: _____
Technologist   Date

Evaluation Criteria

Anatomy Demonstrated

- **AP and AP medial oblique:** Entire foot, including tarsals, metatarsals, and phalanges

Position

AP

- No rotation with tarsals superimposed

AP Medial Oblique

- Third to fifth metatarsals free of superimposition
- Cuboid clearly demonstrated; base of fifth metatarsal seen in profile

Exposure

- Optimal density (brightness) and contrast; no motion
- Soft tissue and sharp bony trabeculation clearly demonstrated

Lateral: Foot

- 18 × 24 cm (8 × 10″) portrait (to foot)

or

- 24 × 30 cm (10 × 12″) portrait for large foot
- Nongrid

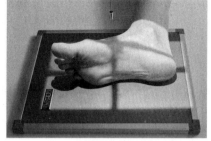

Fig. 4.16 Mediolateral foot.

Position
(Mediolateral)

- Recumbent, on affected side, knee flexed with unaffected leg behind to prevent overrotation
- Place support under affected knee and leg, as needed, to place plantar surface of foot perpendicular to IR for a true lateral

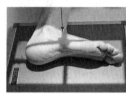

Fig. 4.17 Lateromedial foot.

Lateromedial Projection: May be easier to achieve a true lateral if patient's condition allows this position

Central Ray: CR ⊥, centered to area of base of third metatarsal

SID: 40″ (102 cm)

Collimation: Four sides to skin margins of foot and distal ankle

	cm	kV	mA	Time	mAs	SID	Exposure Indicator
kV Range:		Analog: **60 ± 5 kV**			Digital Systems: **65 ± 5 kV**		
S							
M							
L							

Lower Limb

4

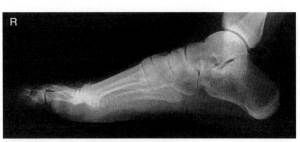

Fig. 4.18 Mediolateral foot.

Competency Check: _____

Technologist   Date

Evaluation Criteria

Anatomy Demonstrated

- Entire foot with ≈1″ (2.5 cm) of distal tibia-fibula

Position

- True lateral with tibiotalar joint open
- Distal metatarsals superimposed

Exposure

- Optimal density (brightness) and contrast; no motion
- Soft tissue and sharp bony trabeculation clearly demonstrated

4

Lower Limb

Weight-Bearing AP and Lateral: Foot

Lateral projection is most common for longitudinal arch (flat feet); AP demonstrates alignment of metatarsals and phalanges. Bilateral projections of both feet are often taken for comparison.

- 24 × 30 cm (10 × 12″) landscape; 35 × 43 cm (14 × 17″) landscape for bilateral study
- Nongrid

Position

- **AP:** Erect, weight evenly distributed on both feet, on one IR
- **Lateral:** Erect, full weight on both feet, vertical IR between feet, standing on blocks, high enough from floor for horizontal CR (R and L feet taken for comparison)

Central Ray:

- **AP:** CR 15° posteriorly, CR to level of base of third metatarsal, midway between feet
- **Lateral:** CR horizontal, to base of third metatarsal

SID: 40″ (102 cm)

Collimation: Collimate to outer skin margins of the feet

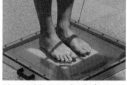

Fig. 4.19 AP—both feet CR 15° posteriorly.

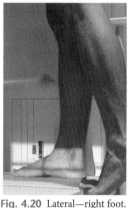

Fig. 4.20 Lateral—right foot.

		Analog: 65 ± 5 kV		Digital Systems: 65 ± 5 kV		
kV Range:						

	cm	kV	mA	Time	mAs	SID	Exposure Indicator
S							
M							
L							

Weight-Bearing AP and Lateral: Foot

Evaluation Criteria

Anatomy Demonstrated

- **AP:** Bilateral feet with soft tissue detail
- **Lateral:** Entire foot with 1″ (2.5 cm) of distal tibia-fibula

Position:

- **AP:** Open tarsometatarsal joints; with approximately equal spacing of second to fourth metatarsals
- **Lateral:** Dorsum to plantar surface demonstrated; heads of metatarsals superimposed

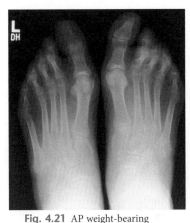

Fig. 4.21 AP weight-bearing bilateral feet.

Competency Check: _____
                    Technologist   Date

Exposure:

- Optimal density (brightness) and contrast
- Soft tissue, cortical margins, and sharp bony trabeculation clearly demonstrated; no motion

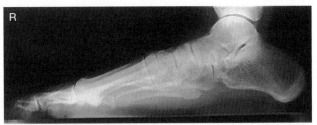

Fig. 4.22 Lateral weight-bearing foot.

Competency Check: _____
                    Technologist   Date

Lower Limb

116

Plantodorsal (Axial): Calcaneus

- 18 × 24 cm (8 × 10″) portrait
- Nongrid (detail screens)
- Lead masking with multiple exposures on same IR

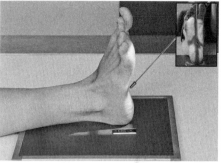

Fig. 4.23 CR 40° to long axis of foot.

Position

- Supine or seated, dorsiflex foot to as near vertical position as possible. If possible, have patient pull on gauze as shown (This may be painful for patient to maintain, so do not delay!)
- Center CR to part, with IR centered to projected CR

Central Ray: CR 40° to long axis of plantar surface (may require more than 40° from vertical if foot is not dorsiflexed a full 90°)

- CR centered to base of third metatarsal, to emerge just distal and inferior to ankle joint
- **Note:** Important to place the calcaneus on the lower aspect of the IR closest to the x-ray tube because of the severe CR angulation

SID: 40″ (102 cm)

Collimation: Collimate closely to region of calcaneus.

kV Range:	Analog: 70 ± 5 kV			Digital Systems: 70 ± 5 kV		
	cm	kV	mA	Time	mAs	SID	Exposure Indicator
S							
M							
L							

Lateral—Mediolateral: Calcaneus

- 18 × 24 cm (8 × 10″) portrait
- Nongrid
- Lead masking with multiple exposures on same IR

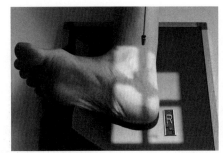

Fig. 4.24 Lateral calcaneus.

Position

- Recumbent, on affected side, knee flexed with unaffected limb behind, to prevent overrotation
- Place support under knee and leg, as needed, for a true lateral
- Dorsiflex foot so that the plantar surface is near 90° to leg, if possible

Central Ray: CR ⊥, to midcalcaneus, 1″ (2.5 cm) inferior to medial malleolus

SID: 40″ (102 cm)

Collimation: Four sides to area of calcaneus; include ankle joint at upper margin

kV Range:		Analog: 60 ± 5 kV			Digital Systems: 70 ± 5 kV		
	cm	kV	mA	Time	mAs	SID	Exposure Indicator
S							
M							
L							

Bontrager Textbook, 9th ed, p. 238.

Plantodorsal (Axial) and Lateral—Mediolateral: Calcaneus

Evaluation Criteria

Anatomy Demonstrated

- **Plantodorsal:** Entire calcaneus from tuberosity to talocalcaneal joint
- **Lateral:** Calcaneus in profile with talus to distal tibia-fibula

Position

- **Plantodorsal:** No rotation with sustentaculum tali in profile medially
- **Lateral:** Partial superimposed talus and open talocalcaneal joint

Exposure

- Density and contrast (brightness) sufficient to faintly visualize distal fibula through talus; no motion
- Sharp bony margins and trabeculation clearly demonstrated

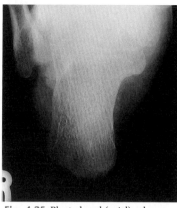

Fig. 4.25 Plantodorsal (axial) calcaneus.

Competency Check: _____
Technologist   Date

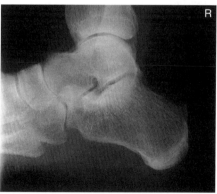

Fig. 4.26 Mediolateral calcaneus.

Competency Check: _____
Technologist   Date

AP: Ankle

- 24 × 30 cm (10 × 12″) portrait
- Nongrid
- Lead masking with multiple exposures on same IR

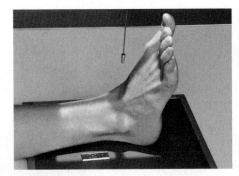

Fig. 4.27 AP ankle.

Position

- Supine or seated on table, leg extended, support under knee
- Align leg and ankle parallel to edge of IR
- True AP, ensure no rotation, long axis of foot is vertical, parallel to CR

Central Ray: CR ⊥, to midway between malleoli

SID: 40″ (102 cm)

Collimation: Collimate to lateral skin margins; include proximal ½ of metatarsals and distal tibia-fibula

		kV Range:	Analog: 60 ± 5 kV		Digital Systems: 70 ± 5 kV		
	cm	kV	mA	Time	mAs	SID	Exposure Indicator
S							
M							
L							

Bontrager Textbook, 9th ed., p. 239.

AP Mortise: Ankle

This is a frontal view of the entire ankle mortise joint and should not be a substitute for the routine AP or 45° oblique ankle.

- 24 × 30 cm (10 × 12″) portrait
- Nongrid
- Lead masking with multiple exposures on same IR

Position

- Supine or seated on table, leg extended, support under knee
- Rotate leg and long axis of foot internally 15°–20° so that **intermalleolar line is parallel to tabletop**

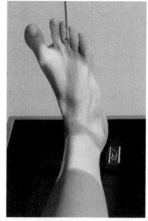

Fig. 4.28 AP, to visualize entire ankle mortise (15°–20° medial rotation).

Central Ray: CR ⊥, to midway between malleoli
SID: 40″ (102 cm)
Collimation: Collimate to lateral skin margins; include distal tibia-fibula and proximal metatarsals in collimation field
Note: The base of the fifth metatarsal is a common fracture site and may be demonstrated in this projection

kV Range:	Analog: 60 ± 5 kV			Digital Systems: 70 ± 5 kV		
	cm	kV	mA	Time	mAs	SID	Exposure Indicator
S							
M							
L							

4

Lower Limb

AP Oblique—45° Medial Rotation: Ankle

- 24 × 30 cm (10 × 12″) portrait
- Nongrid
- Lead masking with multiple exposures on same IR

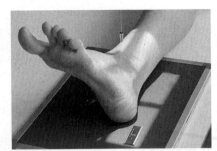

Fig. 4.29 45° AP medial oblique ankle.

Position

- Supine or seated, leg extended, support under knee
- Rotate leg and foot 45° medially (long axis of foot is 45° to IR)

Central Ray: CR ⊥, to midway between the malleoli

SID: 40″ (102 cm)

Collimation: Collimate to ankle region; include proximal metatarsals and distal tibia-fibula

Note: The base of fifth metatarsal is a common fracture site and may be visualized on oblique ankle projections

	cm	kV	mA	Time	mAs	SID	Exposure Indicator
kV Range:		Analog: 60 ± 5 kV			Digital Systems: 70 ± 5 kV		
S							
M							
L							

Bontrager Textbook, 9th ed, p. 241.

AP, AP Mortise, and AP Oblique—45° Medial Rotation: Ankle

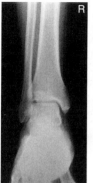 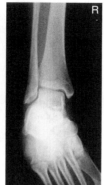 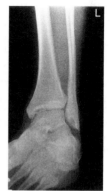

Fig. 4.30 AP ankle. (Courtesy E. Frank, RT[R], FASRT.)

Fig. 4.31 AP mortise ankle.

Fig. 4.32 45° AP medial oblique.

Competency Check: _____

Technologist Date

Evaluation Criteria

Anatomy Demonstrated

- **AP:** Distal $\frac{1}{3}$ of tibia-fibula, lateral and medial malleoli, talus, and proximal metatarsals
- **AP Mortise:** Entire ankle mortise should be open with distal $\frac{1}{3}$ tibia and fibula, lateral and medial malleoli talus and proximal half of metatarsals
- **AP 45° Oblique:** Distal $\frac{1}{3}$ tibia and fibula, malleoli, talus, calcaneus, and proximal half os metatarsals

Position

- **AP:** No rotation with medial mortise joint open and lateral mortise is closed
- **AP Mortise:** Open lateral and medial mortise joint surfaces; malleoli in profile
- **AP 45° Oblique:** Open distal tibiofibular joint, talus, and medial malleolus open with no or only minimal overlap

Exposure

- Density and contrast (brightness) sufficient to faintly visualize distal fibula through talus; no motion
- Soft tissue structures, bony margins and sharp bony trabeculation clearly demonstrated

4

Lower Limb

123

Lateral—Mediolateral or Lateromedial: Ankle

- 24 × 30 cm (10 × 12″) portrait
- Nongrid (detail screens)
- Lead masking with multiple exposures on same IR

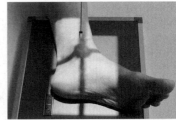

Fig. 4.33 Mediolateral ankle.

Position

- Recumbent, affected side down, affected knee partially flexed
- Dorsiflex foot 90° to leg if patient can tolerate
- Place support under knee as needed for **true lateral** of foot and ankle

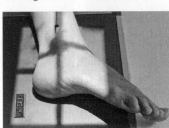

Fig. 4.34 Lateromedial ankle.

Central Ray: CR ⊥, to medial malleolus

Note: May also be taken as a lateromedial projection if patient condition allows, may be easier to achieve a **true lateral**

SID: 40″ (102 cm)

Collimation: Four sides to ankle region; include distal tibia and fibula and proximal metatarsals

kV Range:	Analog: 60 ± 5 kV				Digital Systems: 70 ± 5 kV	
	cm	kV	mA	Time	mAs	SID	Exposure Indicator
S							
M							
L							

Bontrager Textbook, 9th ed, p. 242.

Evaluation Criteria

Anatomy Demonstrated

- Distal $\frac{1}{3}$ of tibia and fibula with lateral view of tarsals, base of fifth metatarsal, navicular and cuboid

Position

- True lateral with no rotation, distal fibula superimposed **over posterior half of tibia**
- Tibiotalar joint open

Exposure

- Density and contrast (brightness) sufficient to faintly visualize distal fibula through talus; no motion
- Sharp bony margins and trabeculation clearly demonstrated

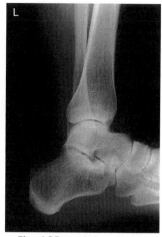

Fig. 4.35 Mediolateral ankle.

Competency Check: _____
    Technologist   Date

4

Lower Limb

125

AP Stress: Ankle
Inversion and Eversion Positions

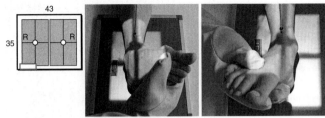

Fig. 4.36 Inversion stress.   Fig. 4.37 Eversion stress.

Warning: Stress must be applied very carefully, either by a long gauze held by the patient or handheld by a qualified person wearing lead gloves and an apron (may require injection of local anesthetic by a physician).
- 24 × 30 cm (10 × 12″) portrait or 35 × 43 cm (14 × 17″) landscape
- Nongrid
- Lead masking with multiple exposures on same IR

Position
- Supine or seated on table, leg extended
- Without rotating leg or ankle (true AP), stress is applied to ankle joint by first turning plantar surface of foot inward (inversion stress), then outward (eversion stress)

Central Ray: CR ⊥, to midway between malleoli
SID: 40″ (102 cm)
Collimation: Collimate to lateral skin margins, including proximal metatarsals and distal tibia-fibula

	cm	kV	mA	Time	mAs	SID	Exposure Indicator
S							
M							
L							

kV Range: Analog: 60 ± 5 kV   Digital Systems: 70 ± 5 kV

Bontrager Textbook, 9th ed, p. 243.

4

Lower Limb

AP: Lower Leg (Tibia-Fibula)

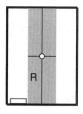

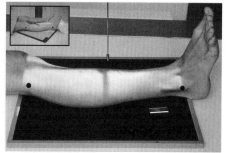

Fig. 4.38 AP lower leg.

- 35 × 43 cm (14 × 17″) portrait; diagonal IR alignment only if needed to include both ankle and knee joints
- Nongrid
- Knee at cathode end to utilize anode heel effect

Position

- Supine, leg extended, ensure no rotation of knee, lower leg, or ankle
- Include ≈3 cm (1–1.5″) minimum beyond knee and ankle joints, considering divergent rays

Central Ray: CR ⊥, to midshaft of lower leg (to mid-IR)

SID: Minimum SID of 40″ (102 cm); may increase to 44–48″ (112–123 cm)

Collimation: On four sides to skin margins to include knee and ankle joints

kV Range:		Analog: 70 ± 5 kV			Digital Systems: 75 ± 5 kV		
	cm	kV	mA	Time	mAs	SID	Exposure Indicator
S							
M							
L							

Lower Limb

4

Mediolateral: Lower Leg (Tibia-Fibula)

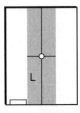

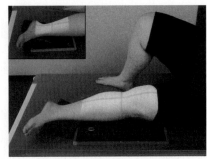

Fig. 4.39 Mediolateral lower leg.

- 35 × 43 cm (14 × 17") portrait; diagonal IR alignment or two separate IRs to include both joints
- Nongrid
- Knee at cathode end (to utilize anode heel effect)

Position
- Recumbent, affected side down
- Place unaffected limb behind patient to prevent overrotation
- Place support under distal portion of affected foot as needed to ensure a **true lateral** position of foot, ankle, and knee
- Ensure that both ankle and knee joints are 1–2" (3–5 cm) from ends of IR

Central Ray: CR ⊥, to midshaft of lower leg (to mid-IR)

SID: Minimum SID of 40" (102 cm); may increase to 44–48" (112–123 cm)

Collimation: On four sides to skin margins to include knee and ankle joints

	cm	kV	mA	Time	mAs	SID	Exposure Indicator
S							
M							
L							

kV Range: Analog: 70 ± 5 kV   Digital Systems: 75 ± 5 kV

Bontrager Textbook, 9th ed, p. 245.

4

Lower Limb

AP and Lateral: Lower Leg (Tibia-Fibula)

Evaluation Criteria

Anatomy Demonstrated

- **AP:** Entire tibia-fibula with ankle and knee joints
- **Lateral:** Entire tibia-fibula with ankle and knee joints

Position

AP

- No rotation, with femoral and tibial condyles in profile
- Slight overlap at both proximal and distal tibiofibular joints

Lateral

- Tibial tuberosity in profile
- Distal fibula overlaps posterior portion of tibia

Exposure

- Near equal density (brightness) and contrast; no motion
- Soft tissue and sharp bony trabeculation clearly demonstrated

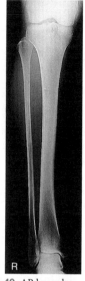

Fig. 4.40 AP lower leg. (Courtesy J. Sanderson, RT.)

Competency Check: _____
Technologist   Date

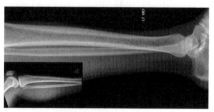

Fig. 4.41 Mediolateral lower leg.

Competency Check: _____
Technologist   Date

AP: Knee

- 24 × 30 cm (10 × 12″) portrait
- Grid >10 cm
- IR <10 cm

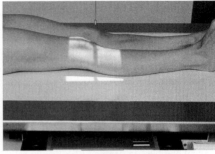

Fig. 4.42 AP knee (CR ⊥, to film for average patient).

Position

- Supine, or seated on table, with leg extended and centered to CR and midline of table or IR
- Rotate leg slightly inward, as needed, to place knee and lower leg into a true AP
- Center IR to CR

Central Ray: CR centered to ½ ″ (1.25 cm) distal to apex of patella

CR Parallel to Articular Facets (Tibial Plateau): Measure distance from ASIS to tabletop (TT) to determine CR angle

- Thin thighs and buttocks (<19 cm ASIS to TT), 3°–5° caudad
- Average thighs and buttocks (19–24 cm), 0°, ⊥ IR
- Thick thighs and buttocks (>24 cm), 3°–5° cephalad

SID: 40″ (102 cm)

Collimation: Sides to skin margins; ends to IR borders

kV Range:		Analog: 65–75 kV				Digital Systems: 75 ± 5 kV	
	cm	kV	mA	Time	mAs	SID	Exposure Indicator
S							
M							
L							

Bontrager Textbook, 9th ed, p. 246.

AP Oblique—Medial and Lateral Rotation: Knee

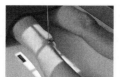

Fig. 4.43 AP 45° medial oblique.

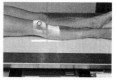

Fig. 4.44 AP 45° lateral oblique.

AP Medial Oblique: Demonstrates fibular head and neck unobscured. (Lateral oblique may also be taken.)

AP Lateral Oblique: Demonstrates medial condyles of the femur and tibia in profile

- 24 × 30 cm (10 × 12″) portrait
- Grid >10 cm
- IR <10 cm

Position

- Semisupine, leg extended and centered to CR and midline of table
- Rotate entire leg, including knee, ankle, and foot, internally 45° for medial oblique, and 45° externally for external oblique
- Center IR to CR

Central Ray:

- CR ⊥, to IR on average patient (see AP Knee)
- CR to midjoint space (½″ or 1.25 cm inferior to patella)

SID: 40″ (102 cm)

Collimation: Sides to skin margins; ends to IR borders

	cm	kV	mA	Time	mAs	SID	Exposure Indicator
kV Range:		Analog: 65–75 kV			Digital Systems: 75 ± 5 kV		
S							
M							
L							

4

Lower Limb

AP and AP Oblique—Medial and Lateral: Knee

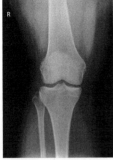

Fig. 4.45 AP knee. (Courtesy Joss Wertz, DO.)

Competency Check: _____
           Technologist   Date

Fig. 4.46 AP medial oblique.

Competency Check: _____
           Technologist   Date

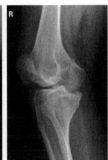

Fig. 4.47 AP lateral oblique. (Courtesy Joss Wertz, DO.)

Competency Check: _____
           Technologist   Date

Evaluation Criteria

Anatomy Demonstrated

- **AP:** Open femorotibial joint space
- **AP Medial Oblique:** Open proximal tibiofibular joint; lateral femoral and tibial condyles in profile
- **AP Lateral Oblique:** Medial femoral and tibial condyles in profile

Position

- **AP:** No rotation is evident by symmetric appearance of femoral and tibial condyles. Medial half of fibular head is superimposed by tibia. Intercondylar eminence is seen
- **AP Medial Oblique:** Proximal tibiofibular joint is open; tibial lateral condyles are demonstrated. Head and neck of fibula and half of patella are seen without superimposition
- **AP Lateral Oblique:** Proximal fibula is superimposed by proximal tibia. Medial condyles of femur and tibia are in profile; Approximately half of patella should be seen free of superimposition by the femur

Exposure

- Optimal density (brightness) and contrast; outline of patella through distal femur; no motion
- Soft tissue and sharp bony trabeculation clearly demonstrated

132

4

Lower Limb

Lateral—Mediolateral: Knee

- 24 × 30 cm (10 × 12″) portrait
- Grid >10 cm
- IR <10 cm

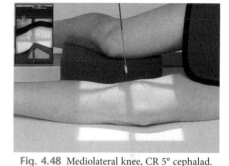

Fig. 4.48 Mediolateral knee, CR 5° cephalad.

Position
- Patient on affected side, knee flexed ≈20°–30°, centered to CR and midline of table or IR
- Unaffected leg and knee placed behind to prevent overrotation
- Place support under affected ankle and foot, if needed, and adjust body rotation as required for a true lateral of knee
- Center IR to CR

Central Ray:
- CR 5°–7° cephalad (if lower leg can be elevated to plane of femur, a perpendicular CR can be used)
- CR centered to ≈1" (2.5 cm) distal to medial epicondyle

SID: 40″ (102 cm)

Collimation: Sides to skin margins; ends to borders of IR

kV Range: Analog: 65–75 kV   Digital Systems: 75 ± 5 kV

	cm	kV	mA	Time	mAs	SID	Exposure Indicator
S							
M							
L							

Evaluation Criteria
Anatomy Demonstrated
- Distal femur, proximal tibia and fibula, and patella in lateral profile
- Patellofemoral and knee joints open

Position
- True lateral with no rotation; femoral condyles superimposed
- Patella in profile and patellofemoral joint open

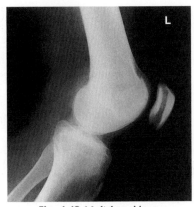

Fig. 4.49 Mediolateral knee.

Competency Check: _____

Technologist   Date

Exposure
- Optimal density (brightness) and contrast; no motion
- Soft tissue (fat pads) and sharp bony trabeculation clearly demonstrated

4

Lower Limb

AP or PA Weight-Bearing Bilateral: Knee

- 35 × 43 cm (14 × 17″) landscape
- Grid

Position
AP
- Erect, standing on step stool or footboard as needed (high enough to lower x-ray tube for horizontal beam)

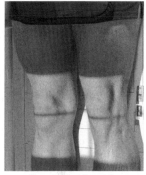

Fig. 4.50 AP weight-bearing—bilateral, CR ⊥ to IR.

- Feet straight ahead, knees straight, weight distributed evenly on both feet. Have patient hold onto table handles for support

Alternative PA: Patient facing the table or IR holder, with knees against table or vertical IR holder, knees flexed ≈20°

Central Ray: CR to midpoint between knee joints, at level of ≈½″ (1.25 cm) distal to apex of patellae

AP: CR horizontal, ⊥ to IR on average patient (see AP Knee)

PA: CR 10° caudad (if knees are flexed ≈20°).

SID: 40″ (102 cm)

Collimation: To bilateral knee joint region including distal femurs and proximal tibia and fibula

kV Range:	Analog: 70 ± 5 kV			Digital Systems: 75 ± 5 kV		
	cm	kV	mA	Time	mAs	SID	Exposure Indicator
S							
M							
L							

Lower Limb

4

PA Axial Weight-Bearing Bilateral: Knee
Rosenberg Method

- 35 × 43 cm (14 × 17″) landscape
- Grid

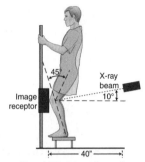

Fig. 4.51 PA axial weight-bearing—CR 10° caudad.

Position
- Patient erect PA
- Weight evenly distributed
- Knees flexed to 45°

Central Ray: 10° caudad to midknee joints— ½″ (1.25 cm) below apex of patella.

SID: 40″ (102 cm)

Collimation: Bilateral knee joint region, including distal femora and proximal tibia

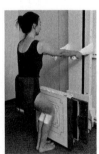

Fig. 4.52 Rosenberg method.

kV Range:	Analog: 70 ± 5 kV				Digital Systems: 75 ± 5 kV	
	cm	kV	mA	Time	mAs	SID	Exposure Indicator
S							
M							
L							

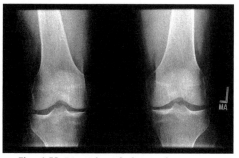

Fig. 4.53 PA axial weight-bearing knees—
Rosenberg method.

Competency Check: _____

              Technologist   Date

Evaluation Criteria

Anatomy Demonstrated
- Distal femur, proximal tibia and fibula, femorotibial joint spaces, and intercondylar fossa

Position
- No rotation of both knees evident by symmetric appearance
- Articular facets in profile

Exposure
- Optimal density (brightness) and contrast; no motion
- Sharp bony trabeculation clearly demonstrated

Lower Limb

4

137

PA and AP Axial ("Tunnel Views"): Intercondylar Fossa
Camp Coventry and Holmblad Methods

- 18 × 24 cm (8 × 10") portrait
- Grid

Position:
- Camp Coventry method: Prone, knee flexed 40°–50°, large support under ankle
- Holmblad method: Kneeling on x-ray table or partially standing
- Knee centered to CR
- IR centered to projected CR

Central Ray:
- **Camp Coventry method:** CR 40°–50° caudad (⊥ to lower leg), centered to knee joint, to emerge at distal margin of patella

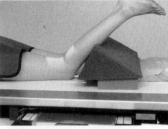

Fig. 4.54 PA axial projection (Camp Coventry).

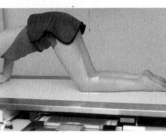

Fig. 4.55 Alternative Holmblad method:
– Patient kneeling, leans forward 20°–30°
– CR ⊥ to IR

- **Holmblad method:** CR ⊥ to lower leg to midpopliteal crease

SID: 40" (102 cm)

Collimation: Four sides to area of interest

	cm	kV	mA	Time	mAs	SID	Exposure Indicator
S							
M							
L							

kV Range: Analog: 70 ± 5 kV   Digital Systems: 75 ± 5 kV

Bontrager Textbook, 9th ed, p. 253.

Lower Limb

4

PA: Patella

- 18 × 24 cm (8 × 10") portrait
- Grid

Position
- Prone, knee centered to CR and midline of table or IR

Fig. 4.56 PA patella.

- If patella area is painful, place pad under thigh and leg to prevent direct pressure on patella
- Rotate anterior knee approximately 5° internally or as needed to place an imaginary line between the epicondyles parallel to the plane of the IR
- Center IR to CR

Central Ray: CR ⊥, centered to central patella region (at midpopliteal crease)

SID: 40" (102 cm)

Collimation: To area of patella and knee joint

kV Range:	Analog: 75 ± 5 kV (Increase 4–6 kV from PA Knee)				Digital Systems: 75 ± 5 kV		
	cm	kV	mA	Time	mAs	SID	Exposure Indicator
S							
M							
L							

Lateral—Mediolateral: Patella

- 18 × 24 cm (8 × 10")
  portrait
- Nongrid (detail
  screens—may use
  grid on large patient)

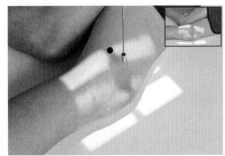

Fig. 4.57 Mediolateral patella.

Position
- Recumbent on affected side, opposite knee, and leg behind to
  prevent overrotation
- Flex knee only 5°–10° to prevent separation of fractured
  fragments, if present
- Patellofemoral joint area centered to CR and midline of IR

Central Ray: CR ⊥, centered to midpatellofemoral joint

SID: 40" (102 cm)

Collimation: To area of knee joint, patella, and patellofemoral joint

kV Range:		Analog: 70 ± 6 kV			Digital Systems: 75 ± 5 kV		
	cm	kV	mA	Time	mAs	SID	Exposure Indicator
S							
M							
L							

Bontrager Textbook, 9th ed, p. 257.

PA Axial: Intercondylar Fossa
PA and Lateral: Patella

Evaluation Criteria
Anatomy Demonstrated
- **PA Axial:** Intercondylar fossa, femoral condyles, tibial plateaus, and intercondylar eminence
- **PA:** Knee joint and patella outline through distal femur
- **Lateral:** Patella, patellofemoral joint, and femorotibial joint demonstrated in profile

Position
- **PA Axial:** No rotation evidenced by symmetric distal femoral condyles and intercondylar eminence centered
- **PA:** No rotation, femoral condyles appear symmetric; patella appears centered to femur
- **Lateral:** Patella in profile and patellofemoral joint open

Exposure
- Optimal density (brightness) and contrast; no motion
- Soft tissue and sharp bony trabeculation clearly demonstrated

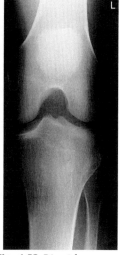

Fig. 4.58 PA axial—intercondylar fossa projection.

Competency
Check: _____
        Technologist   Date

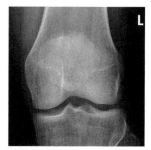

Fig. 4.59 PA patella.
(Courtesy Joss Wertz, DO.)

Competency
Check: _____
Technologist   Date

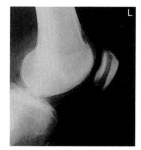

Fig. 4.60 Lateral patella.

Competency
Check: _____
    Technologist   Date

Tangential—Axial: Patella
Merchant Bilateral Method

- 18 × 24 cm (8 × 10″) landscape or 35 × 43 cm (14 × 17″) landscape for large knees
- Nongrid
- Adjustable leg and IR-holding device required

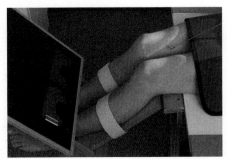

Fig. 4.61 Bilateral tangential.

Position
- Supine with knees flexed 40° on leg supports (important for patient to be comfortable with legs totally relaxed to prevent patellae from being drawn into intercondylar sulcus)
- Place IR on supports against legs about 12″ (30 cm) distal to patellae, perpendicular to CR

Central Ray:
- CR 30° caudad from horizontal (30° from long axis of femora)
- CR to midpoint between patellae

SID: 48–72″ (123–183 cm) greater SID reduces magnification

Collimation: To bilateral patellae

	cm	kV	mA	Time	mAs	SID	Exposure Indicator
kV Range:	Analog: 70 ± 5 kV			Digital Systems: 75 ± 5 kV			
S							
M							
L							

Bontrager Textbook, 9th ed, p. 258.

4

Lower Limb

Tangential—Axial (Prone): Patella
Settegast and Hughston Methods

Generally taken bilaterally for comparison purposes.

- 24 × 30 cm (10 × 12″) landscape
- Nongrid
- Lead masking with multiple exposures on same IR

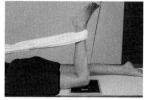

Fig. 4.62 Settegast:
– Knee flexed 90°
– CR 15°–20° to lower leg

4

Position

- **Settegast:** Prone, knee flexed 90°
- **Hughston:** Prone, knee flexed between 50° and 60° from full extension
- Use long gauze or tape for patient to hold leg in position; for Hughston method, may support foot on supporting device (not collimator)

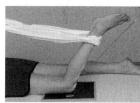

Fig. 4.63 Hughston:
– Knee flexed 50°–60°
– CR 45° cephalad
Warning: Possible hot collimator, use pad.

Lower Limb

Central Ray: CR centered to mid-patellofemoral joint
Settegast: CR 15°–20° cephalad to long axis of leg (knee flexed 90°)
Hughston: CR 45° cephalad to long axis of leg (knee flexed 50°–60°)
SID: 40–48″ (102–123 cm)
Collimate: Closely to patella region

kV Range:	Analog: 70 ± 5 kV			Digital Systems: 75 ± 5 kV		

	cm	kV	mA	Time	mAs	SID	Exposure Indicator
S							
M							
L							

Superoinferior Sitting Tangential: Patella
Hobbs Modification

Generally taken bilaterally on one IR for comparison purposes

- 35 × 43 cm (14 × 17″) landscape or 18 × 24 cm (8 × 10″), landscape (unilateral)
- Nongrid

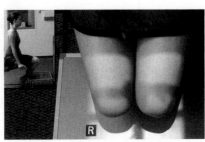

Fig. 4.64 Tangential superoinferior (Hobbs modification).

Position
- Patient seated
- Knees flexed with feet placed under chair
- IR placed on footstool

Central Ray: Perpendicular to IR (tangential to patellofemoral joint) centered to midway between patellofemoral joints

SID: 48–50″ (123–128 cm)

Collimation: Bilateral knee joint region, distal femora, and patella

kV Range:	Analog: 70 ± 5 kV			Digital Systems: 75 ± 5 kV		
	cm	kV	mA	Time	mAs	SID	Exposure Indicator
S							
M							
L							

Bontrager Textbook, 9th ed, p. 261.

Superoinferior Sitting Tangential (Bilateral): Patella

Hobbs Modification

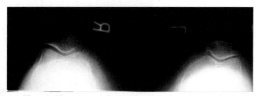

Fig. 4.65 Superoinferior tangential sitting method.

Competency Check: _____

Technologist   Date

Evaluation Criteria

Anatomy Demonstrated

- Tangential view of patella
- Patellofemoral joint space open

Position

- Separation of patella and intercondylar sulcus
- Patellofemoral joint open

Exposure

- Optimal density (brightness) and contrast; no motion
- Soft tissue and sharp bony trabeculation clearly demonstrated

AP: Lower Limb (Pediatric)

- Size determined by patient size
- Nongrid (detail screen)

Note: If foot is specific area of interest, AP and lateral projections of foot only may be required.

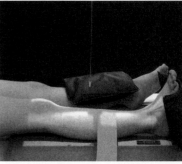

Fig. 4.66 AP lower limb.

Position—Shield Radiosensitive Tissues

- Supine, include entire limb, shield over pelvic area
- A second IR of pelvis and/or proximal femur may be required (see Chapter 16 in the Bontrager textbook)
- Immobilize arms and unaffected leg with sandbags
- Use parental assistance only if necessary; provide lead gloves and apron

Central Ray: CR ⊥, centered to midlimb (mid-IR)
SID: 40″ (102 cm)
Collimation: Four sides to area of interest

kV Range:		Analog: 55–70 kV			Digital Systems: 60–75 kV		
	cm	kV	mA	Time	mAs	SID	Exposure Indicator
S							
M							
L							

Lateral: Lower Limb (Pediatric)

- Size determined by patient size
- Nongrid (detail screen)

Note: If foot is specific area of interest, AP and lateral projections of foot only may also be required.

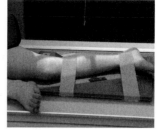

Fig. 4.67 Lateral lower limb (see *Note*).

Position—Shield Radiosensitive Tissues

- Semisupine, include entire limb, shield over pelvic area
- Immobilize arms and unaffected leg with sandbags, as needed
- Abduct (frog leg) affected limb into lateral position, immobilize with tape or compression band (Do not attempt in patients with hip trauma or hip disease)
- If parental assistance is necessary, provide lead gloves and apron

Central Ray: CR ⊥, centered to midlimb (mid-IR)

SID: 40″ (102 cm)

Collimation: Four sides to area of interest

kV Range:	Analog: 55–70 kV			Digital Systems: 60–75 kV		

	cm	kV	mA	Time	mAs	SID	Exposure Indicator
S							
M							
L							

AP and Mediolateral: Foot (Pediatric)
Congenital Clubfoot—Kite Method

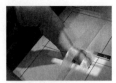

Fig. 4.68 AP foot.

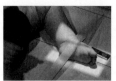

Fig. 4.69 Mediolateral foot.

- 18 × 24 cm (8 × 10″) portrait
- Nongrid (detail screens)

Note: With **Kite method,** no attempt is made to straighten foot when placing on IR. The foot is held or immobilized for a frontal and side view (AP and lateral projections) 90° from each other. Both feet are generally imaged for comparison.

Position
- **AP:** Elevate patient on support, flex knee, foot on IR
- **Lateral:** Patient and/or leg on side, affected side down, use tape or compression band

Central Ray
- **AP:** CR ⊥, to IR, directed to midtarsals (Kite recommends no angle)
- **Lateral:** CR ⊥, centered to proximal metatarsal area

SID: 40″ (102 cm)

Collimation: Closely on four sides to area of foot

	cm	kV	mA	Time	mAs	SID	Exposure Indicator
kV Range:		Analog: 55–70 kV			Digital Systems: 60–75 kV		
S							
M							
L							

Bontrager Textbook, 9th ed, p. 634.

Chapter 5

Femur and Pelvic Girdle

5

Femur and Pelvic Girdle

(R) Routine, (S) Special

149

Radiation Protection

Accurate gonadal shielding for pelvis and hip examinations is especially critical because of the proximity of radiation-sensitive tissues (proximal femurs, gonads, noninvolved portions of the pelvis) to the primary x-ray beam. But shielding must not interfere with clinical intent of radiographic study.

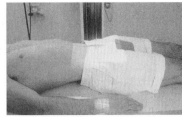

Fig. 5.1 Male gonadal shielding.

Male Shielding: Gonadal shields should be used on pelvis and hip procedures for all males. Contact shields should be placed over the testes, with the upper edge of the shield placed at the inferior margin of the symphysis pubis.

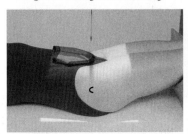

Fig. 5.2 Female ovarian shielding (superior borders at or slightly above level of ASISs and lower border just above pubis).

Female Shielding: For AP and "frog-leg" laterals of the hips, specially shaped ovarian shields can be carefully placed over the area of the ovaries without obscuring essential anatomy, as shown. This should be done on all females. These ovarian shields, however, may obscure essential anatomy on certain pelvic examinations. Departmental policy regarding shielding and kV range to be used should be determined.

kV Range: A higher kV range (80 to 90 kV) with lower mAs may be used for examinations of the hips and pelvis of adults to reduce the total radiation dose to the patient.

Close collimation to the area of interest is important for all procedures, including the hips and pelvis, even with gonadal shields. (See Appendix A for further explanation.)

Localization Methods for Femoral Head and Neck

First Method: Location of the femoral head and neck regions can be accurately determined by first drawing an imaginary line between two landmarks, the **ASIS** and the **symphysis pubis.** The midpoint of this line is determined, from which a perpendicular imaginary line is drawn to locate the head and/or neck. The femoral head (A) is approximately 1.5″ (4 cm) down on this line. The midfemoral neck (B) is approximately 2.5″ (6–7 cm) down, as shown in the photo below.

Second Method: A second method for locating the femoral neck (B) is ≈1–2″ (2.5–5 cm) medial to the ASIS at the level of the proximal or upper margin of the symphysis pubis, which is 3–4″ (8–10 cm) distal to the ASIS.

Method one:
Head–1.5″
(4 cm)
Neck–2.5″
(6–7 cm)

Method two:
1–2″
(3–5 cm)

3–4″
(8–10 cm)

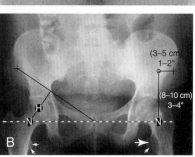

Femur and Pelvic Girdle

Fig. 5.3 A, Femoral head. **B,** Femoral neck.

AP: Femur

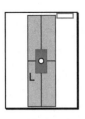

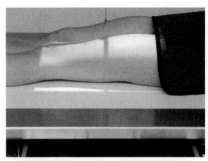

Fig. 5.4 AP mid- and distal femur.

- 35 × 43 cm (14 × 17″) portrait
- Grid
- Hip at cathode end (anode heel effect)

Note: For adults, a second smaller IR of either the hip or the knee should be taken on trauma patients to demonstrate both knee and hip joints to rule out possible fractures.

Position

- Supine, femur centered to midline of table or grid IR
- Rotate entire lower limb internally ≈5° for AP of midfemur and distal femur, and 15° internally for true AP to include hip
- Lower border of IR ≈5 cm (2″) below knee to include knee joint adequately (see AP Unilateral Hip for proximal femur, p. 153)
- **Shield radiosensitive tissues** for both male and female

Central Ray: CR ⊥ to femur, to mid-IR

SID: 40″ (102 cm)

Collimation: Long, narrow collimation to femur area

	cm	kV	mA	Time	mAs	SID	Exposure Indicator
S							
M							
L							

kV Range: Analog: 75 ± 5 kV   Digital Systems: 80 ± 5 kV

Bontrager Textbook, 9th ed, p. 276.

Lateral: Femur

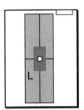

Warning: Take horizontal beam lateral if fracture is suspected.

- 35 × 43 cm (14 × 17″) portrait
- Grid
- Hip at cathode end (anode heel effect)

Note: For adults, take a second, smaller IR of lateral hip or lateral knee if both joints are areas of interest.

Position

- Lateral recumbent, with unaffected leg placed behind to prevent over-rotation
- Include sufficient amount of either knee or hip at one end of IR.
- Flex affected knee ≈45°, and align femur to midline of table
- Shield radiosensitive tissues when possible

Central Ray: CR ⊥ femur, to mid-IR

SID: 40″ (102 cm)

Collimation: Long, narrow collimation to femur area

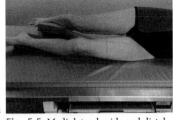

Fig. 5.5 Mediolateral mid- and distal femur.

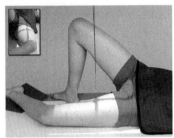

Fig. 5.6 Mediolateral mid- and proximal femur.

kV Range:		Analog: 75 ± 5 kV		Digital Systems: 80 ± 5 kV			
	cm	kV	mA	Time	mAs	SID	Exposure Indicator
S							
M							
L							

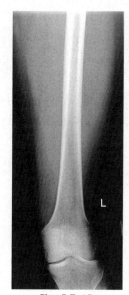

Fig. 5.7 AP.

Competency Check: _____

Technologist   Date

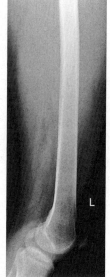

Fig. 5.8 Lateral.

Competency Check: _____

Technologist   Date

Evaluation Criteria

Anatomy Demonstrated

- **AP and Lateral:** Distal ⅔ of femur, including knee joint

Position

- **AP:** No rotation, femoral and tibial condyles appear symmetric in size and shape
- **Lateral:** True lateral, femoral condyles appear superimposed

Exposure

AP and Lateral

- Optimal density (brightness) and contrast
- Fine trabecular markings; no motion

Horizontal Beam Lateral:
Mid- and Distal Femur (Trauma)

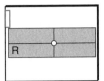

- 35 × 43 cm (14 × 17″) portrait (to long axis of femur)
- Portable grid

Note: For proximal femur injuries, perform axiolateral (Danelius-Miller method) hip.

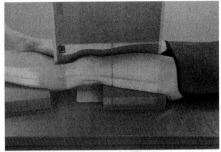

Fig. 5.9 Horizontal beam trauma projection (mid- and distal femur).

Position
- Without moving trauma patient from the supine position, gently lift injured leg, and place support under knee and leg
- Place vertical IR between legs, as far superiorly as possible, but include knee distally. Use tape to hold grid IR in position
- **Shield radiosensitive tissues** for both male and female

Central Ray: CR horizontal beam, ⊥ to femur to midpoint of IR
SID: 40″ (102 cm)
Collimation: Closely to four sides to area of interest

kV Range: Analog: 75 ± 5 kV   Digital Systems: 80 ± 5 kV

	cm	kV	mA	Time	mAs	SID	Exposure Indicator
S							
M							
L							

Femur and Pelvic Girdle

5

AP Bilateral: Proximal Femora (Hips)

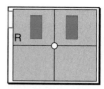

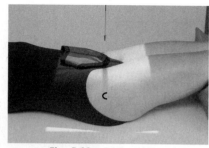

Warning: Do not attempt to rotate leg if fracture is suspected. Perform "as is" bilateral hips for comparison purposes.

Fig. 5.10 AP bilateral hips.

Note: For AP pelvis centering, see p. 273 in Bontrager textbook.

- 35 × 43 cm (14 × 17″) landscape
- Grid

Position

- Supine, aligned and centered to CR and IR, both legs extended and equally rotated internally 15°–20° (see *Warning* above)
- Ensure no rotation of pelvis (bilateral ASISs the same distances from tabletop). Support under knees for patient comfort
- Center IR to CR. **Shield radiosensitive tissues** (males and females)

Central Ray: CR ⊥, to midpoint between femoral heads (which is about 2 cm or 1″ superior to symphysis pubis)

SID: 40″ (102 cm)

Collimation: To pelvic and hip borders

Respiration: Suspend during exposure

kV Range:	Analog: 80 ± 5 kV			Digital Systems: 85 ± 5 kV			
	cm	kV	mA	Time	mAs	SID	Exposure Indicator
S							
M							
L							

Bontrager Textbook, 9th ed, p. 279.

Femur and Pelvic Girdle

AP Unilateral: Proximal Femur (Hip)

Warning: For possible fractured hip, perform AP bilateral hips (preceding page) for comparison purposes.

- 24 × 30 cm (10 × 12″) portrait
- Grid

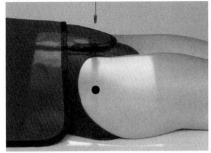

Fig. 5.11 AP hip—CR to femoral neck.

Position

- Supine, leg extended and rotated internally 15°–20° (nontrauma)
- Center femoral neck to CR; support may be placed under knees for patient comfort
- Center IR to CR; **shield radiosensitive tissues** (males and females)

Central Ray: CR ⊥ IR, directed to 1–2″ (2.5–5 cm) distal to mid-femoral neck (to include all of orthopedic appliance of hip, if present)

SID: 40″ (102 cm)

Collimation: Four sides to area of interest

Respiration: Suspend during exposure

| kV Range: | Analog: 80 ± 5 kV | | | Digital Systems: 80 ± 5 kV | | |

	cm	kV	mA	Time	mAs	SID	Exposure Indicator
S							
M							
L							

Femur and Pelvic Girdle

5

AP Unilateral: Proximal Femur (Hip)

Evaluation Criteria

Anatomy Demonstrated

- Proximal ⅓ of femur and adjacent parts of pelvic girdle
- Orthopedic appliance in entirety

Position

- Greater trochanter, femoral head and neck in profile
- Lesser trochanter not visible or minimally only

Exposure

- Optimal density (brightness) and contrast
- Sharp trabecular markings clearly demonstrated; no motion

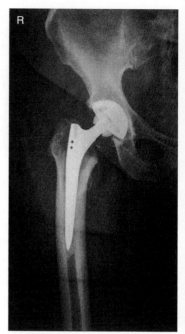

Fig. 5.12 AP hip. (Copyright Getty Images/DieterMeyrl.)

Competency Check: _____

                    Technologist   Date

Unilateral Frog-Leg: Lateral Hip (Nontrauma)
Modified Cleaves Method

Warning: Do **not** attempt with possible fracture of hip area.

- 24 × 30 cm (10 × 12″) landscape
- Grid

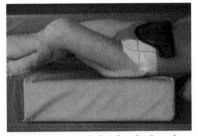

Fig. 5.13 Right hip frog-leg lateral (for femoral neck).

Position

- Patient supine
- For femoral neck, flex affected knee and hip, and abduct femur 45° from vertical*
- For femoral head, acetabulum, and proximal femoral shaft, oblique patient 35°–45° toward affected side and abduct leg to tabletop, if possible. Center hip and neck area to CR

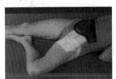

Fig. 5.14 For femoral head and acetabulum and proximal femoral shaft.

- Center IR to CR. **Shield radiosensitive tissues** (male and female)

Central Ray: CR ⊥, to midfemoral neck (see localization methods on p. 151)

SID: 40″ (102 cm)

Collimation: To proximal femur and hip

Respiration: Suspend during exposure

*Less abduction of femora of only 20°–30° from vertical provides for the least foreshortening of femoral neck.

| kV Range: | Analog: 80 ± 5 kV | | | Digital Systems: 80 ± 5 kV | | |

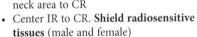

	cm	kV	mA	Time	mAs	SID	Exposure Indicator
S							
M							
L							

Femur and Pelvic Girdle

5

AP Bilateral Frog-Leg: Hips (Nontrauma)
Modified Cleaves Method

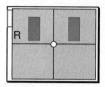

Warning: Do **not** attempt with possible fracture of hip areas.

- 35 × 43 cm (14 × 17") landscape
- Grid

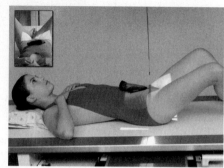

Fig. 5.15 Bilateral frog-leg (for comparison).

Position

- Supine, centered to CR and IR, flex hips and knees and **abduct both femora equally** 40°–45° from vertical,* if possible, with plantar surfaces of feet together
- Ensure **no rotation** of pelvis (ASISs equal distance from table)
- Center IR to CR, **shield radiosensitive tissues** (male and female)

Central Ray: CR ⊥ to IR, to level of femoral heads (≈7–8 cm or 3" inferior to level of ASISs)

SID: 40" (102 cm)

Collimation: On four sides to anatomy of interest

Respiration: Suspend during exposure

*Less abduction of femora of only 20°–30° from vertical provides for the least foreshortening of femoral neck.

	kV Range:	Analog: **80 ± 5 kV**		Digital Systems: **85 ± 5 kV**		

	cm	kV	mA	Time	mAs	SID	Exposure Indicator
S							
M							
L							

Bontrager Textbook, 9th ed., p. 280.

AP Bilateral Frog-Leg: Hips (Nontrauma)

**Evaluation
Criteria**
Anatomy
Demonstrated
- Femoral heads
  and necks,
  acetabulum,
  and
  trochanteric
  anatomy

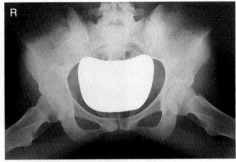

Fig. 5.16 AP bilateral frog-leg.

Position
- No rotation
  evident by
  symmetry of
  pelvic bones
- Lesser trochanters equal in size
- Minimal distortion of femoral neck
- Greater trochanters superimposed over femoral necks

Exposure
- Optimal density (brightness) and contrast
- Sharp trabecular markings clearly demonstrated; no motion

Competency Check:

Technologist

Date

5

Femur and Pelvic Girdle

Axiolateral Inferosuperior: Lateral Hip (Trauma)
Danelius-Miller Method

Warning: Do not attempt to rotate leg internally on initial trauma examination.

- 24 × 30 cm (10 × 12″) landscape (lengthwise to long axis of femur)
- Portable grid

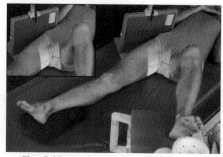

Fig. 5.17 Axiolateral trauma hip (pad under foot).

Position

- Supine, no rotation of pelvis
- Flex and elevate unaffected knee and hip and provide support
- Rotate affected leg internally 15° **unless contraindicated by possible hip fracture**
- Place vertical grid IR against side just superior to iliac crest with plane of IR perpendicular to CR

Central Ray: CR horizontal, perpendicular to femoral neck area and IR (see "hip localization methods" in chapter introduction)

SID: 40″ (102 cm)

Collimation: On four sides to proximal femur area

Respiration: Suspend during exposure

kV Range:	Analog: 80 ± 5 kV			Digital Systems: 90 ± 5 kV		

	cm	kV	mA	Time	mAs	SID	Exposure Indicator
S							
M							
L							

Bontrager Textbook, 9th ed, p. 286.

Axiolateral Inferosuperior: Lateral Hip (Trauma)
Danelius-Miller Method

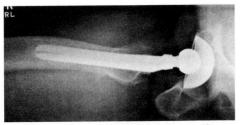

Fig. 5.18 Axiolateral hip. (Courtesy Ferlic Filters, White Bear Lake, Minnesota.)

Competency Check: _____

Technologist   Date

Evaluation Criteria

Anatomy Demonstrated
- Entire femoral head and neck, trochanters, and acetabulum
- Orthopedic appliance in entirety

Position
- Femoral head, neck, and acetabulum demonstrated with little superimposition of opposite hip
- No grid lines visible on radiograph
- Minimal distortion of femoral neck

Exposure
- Optimal density (brightness) and contrast
- Sharp trabecular markings clearly seen; no motion

Femur and Pelvic Girdle

AP: Pelvis

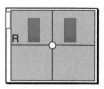

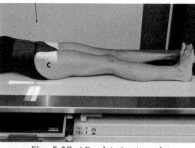

Fig. 5.19 AP pelvis (entire pelvis centered to IR).

To include proximal femora, pelvic girdle, sacrum, and coccyx

Warning: Do not attempt to rotate legs if fractures involving hips are suspected.

Note: For bilateral hips centering, see p. 156.

- 35 × 43 cm (14 × 17″) landscape
- Grid

Position

- Supine, pelvis centered to centerline, legs extended
- Both feet, knees, and legs equally rotated internally 15°–20° (secure with tape, if necessary). Support under knees for comfort
- Ensure no rotation of pelvis (ASISs equal distance from TT)
- Center IR to CR (include entire pelvis). **Shield radiosensitive tissues** (if it does not compromise study)

Central Ray: CR ⊥, midway between ASISs and symphysis pubis (approximately 5 cm or 2″ distal to level of ASISs)

SID: 40″ (102 cm)

Collimation: On four sides to include entire pelvis

Respiration: Suspend during exposure

kV Range:	Analog: 80 ± 5 kV			Digital Systems: 85 ± 5 kV			
	cm	kV	mA	Time	mAs	SID	Exposure Indicator
S							
M							
L							

Bontrager Textbook, 9th ed, p. 279.

AP: Pelvis

Evaluation Criteria

Anatomy Demonstrated

- Pelvic girdle, L5, sacrum, coccyx, and proximal femora
- Orthopedic appliance in entirety (if present)

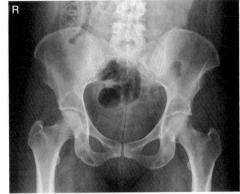

Fig. 5.20 AP pelvis.

Competency Check: _____
Technologist   Date

Position

- Lesser trochanters generally not visible (nontrauma)
- **No rotation** evident by symmetry of ilia and obturator foramina

Exposure

- Optimal density (brightness) and contrast visualizing L5 and sacrum and margins of femoral heads and acetabula
- Soft tissue and sharp trabecular markings clearly demonstrated; no motion

5

Femur and Pelvic Girdle

AP Axial (Inlet and Outlet): Pelvis

- 35 × 43 cm (14 × 17″) landscape
- Grid

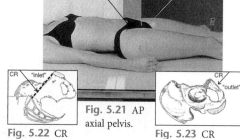

Fig. 5.21 AP axial pelvis.

Fig. 5.22 CR 40° caudal for **inlet.**

Fig. 5.23 CR **cephalad 20°–35° for males** and **30°–45° for females—outlet.**

Position
- Supine, patient centered to centerline
- No rotation of pelvis (ASISs the same distance from tabletop)
- Center IR to projected CR. Gonadal shielding may not be possible without obscuring essential anatomy

Central Ray:
- **Inlet:** CR 40° caudal to level of ASISs, male and female
- **Outlet** (Taylor method): CR: male, 20°–35° cephalad; female, 30°–45° cephalad centered 1–2″ (2.5–5 cm) inferior to symphysis pubis or greater trochanters

SID: 40″ (102 cm)

Collimation: Four sides to area of interest

Respiration: Suspend during exposure

		kV Range:	Analog: **80 ± 5 kV**		Digital Systems: **85 ± 5 kV**	

	cm	kV	mA	Time	mAs	SID	Exposure Indicator
S							
M							
L							

Bontrager Textbook, 9th ed, pp. 281–282.

Femur and Pelvic Girdle

5

AP Axial (Inlet and Outlet): Pelvis

Evaluation Criteria

Anatomy Demonstrated

- **Inlet:** Pelvic ring or inlet in its entirety
- **Outlet:** Superior/inferior rami of pubis and ramus of ischium

Position

- **Inlet:** Ischial spines are demonstrated and equal in size; pelvic ring; no rotation
- **Outlet:** Obturator foramina are equal in size; anterior/ inferior pelvic bones; no rotation

Exposure

- Optimal density (brightness) and contrast; no motion
- Body and superior rami of pubis demonstrated

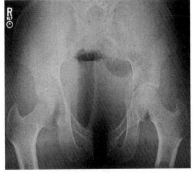

Fig. 5.24 AP axial inlet projection.

Competency Check: _____
Technologist   Date

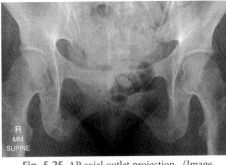

Fig. 5.25 AP axial outlet projection. (Image courtesy Joss Wertz, DO.)

Competency Check: _____
Technologist   Date

- Superimposed anterior and posterior portions of pelvic ring
- Bony margins and trabecular markings appear sharp

5

Femur and Pelvic Girdle

Posterior Oblique: Acetabulum
Judet Method

Note: Both sides are generally imaged for comparison, either both for upside or both for downside.

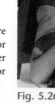

Fig. 5.26 Downside acetabulum.

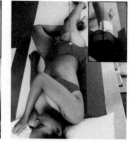

Fig. 5.27 Upside acetabulum.

- 24 × 30 cm (10 × 12″) portrait or 35 × 43 cm (14 × 17″) landscape (if both hips must be seen on each projection)
- Grid

Position
- Patient in 45° posterior oblique position, centered for either upside or downside hip joint (dependent on anatomy of interest)
- Place 45° support under elevated side, position arms and legs as shown to maintain this position

Central Ray:
- **Downside:** CR ⊥ to 2″ (5 cm) distal and 2″ (5 cm) medial to downside ASIS
- **Upside:** CR ⊥ to 2″ (5 cm) distal to upside ASIS

SID: 40″ (102 cm)
Collimation: Four sides to area of interest
Respiration: Suspend during exposure

kV Range:	Analog: **80 ± 5 kV**	Digital Systems: **85 ± 5 kV**

	cm	kV	mA	Time	mAs	SID	Exposure Indicator
S							
M							
L							

Bontrager Textbook, 9th ed, p. 283.

Posterior Oblique: Acetabulum
Judet Method

Evaluation Criteria

Anatomy Demonstrated

- **Downside:** Anterior rim of acetabulum, posterior ilioischial column and iliac wing demonstrated
- **Upside:** Posterior rim of acetabulum, anterior iliopubic column and obturator foramen demonstrated

Position

- **Downside:** Iliac wing elongated and obturator foramen closed
- **Upside:** Iliac wing foreshortened and obturator foramen open

Exposure

- Optimal density (brightness) and contrast
- Bony margins and trabecular markings are sharp; no motion

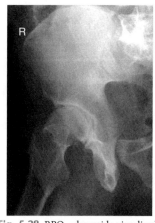

Fig. 5.28 RPO—downside visualized.

Competency Check: _____

Technologist   Date

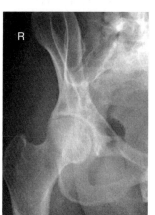

Fig. 5.29 LPO—upside visualized.

Competency Check: _____

Technologist   Date

5

Femur and Pelvic Girdle

PA Axial Oblique: Acetabulum
Teufel Method

Both sides are generally imaged for comparison.
- 24 × 30 cm (10 × 12")
  portrait
- Grid

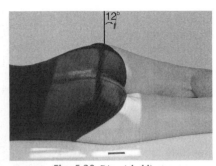

Fig. 5.30 PA axial oblique.

Position
- Patient semiprone; affected side down
- Rotate body 35°–40° anterior oblique

Central Ray:
- CR 12° cephalad
- When anatomy of interest is downside, direct CR ⊥ at 1" (2.5 cm) superior to level of greater trochanter; ≈2" (5 cm) lateral to the midsagittal plane

SID: 40" (102 cm)

Collimation: Region of acetabulum and proximal femur

		kV Range:	Analog: 70–80 kV		Digital Systems: 80 ± 5 kV		
	cm	kV	mA	Time	mAs	SID	Exposure Indicator
S							
M							
L							

Bontrager Textbook, 9th ed, p. 284.

Evaluation Criteria

Anatomy Demonstrated
- Superoposterior wall of the acetabulum

Position
- Fovea capitis with the femoral head in profile
- Obturator foramen open

Exposure
- Optimal density (brightness) and contrast; no motion
- Bony margins and sharp trabecular markings clearly seen

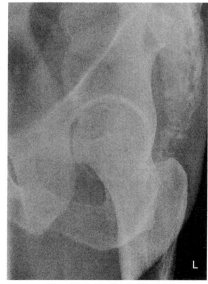

Fig. 5.31 PA axial oblique.

Competency Check: _____

Technologist   Date

5

Femur and Pelvic Girdle

AP and Lateral: Hips and Pelvis (Pediatric)

Warning: Do not attempt frog-leg lateral with possible hip pathology unless so indicated by a physician after review of AP pelvis radiograph.

- Size determined by patient size; IR landscape
- Grid >10 cm

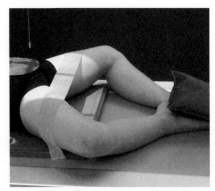

Fig. 5.32 Frog-leg lateral hips.

Position (AP and Lateral)

- Supine, pelvis centered to CR and to IR; **use gonadal shields on both male and female** (Use ovarian shield of appropriate size for female, ensuring that it does not cover hip areas)
- Immobilize arms and upper body with sandbags, tape, or compression band, as needed

AP: Extend legs, and internally rotate 15°

Frog-Leg Lateral: Flex knees and hips, place soles of feet together and abduct both legs, and secure with tape and sandbags

Central Ray: CR ⊥, centered to level of hips

SID: 40″ (102 cm)

Collimation: To pelvic margins

Respiration: Full inspiration if crying

| | | kV Range: | Analog: 60–65 kV | | | Digital Systems: 65–75 kV | |

	cm	kV	mA	Time	mAs	SID	Exposure Indicator
S							
M							
L							

172   Bontrager Textbook, 9th ed, p. 635.

5

Femur and Pelvic Girdle

Chapter 6

Vertebral Column

6

Vertebral Column

(R) Routine, (S) Special

Vertebral Column

Intervertebral Foramina and Zygapophyseal Joints

Certain lateral and oblique projections best demonstrate these important foramina and joints of the spine as follows:

	Zygapophyseal Joints	Intervertebral Foramina
Cervical spine	Lateral position	45° anterior oblique (side closest to IR)
Thoracic spine	70° anterior oblique (side closest to IR)	Lateral position
Lumbar spine	45° posterior oblique (side closest to IR)	Lateral position

Topographic Landmarks

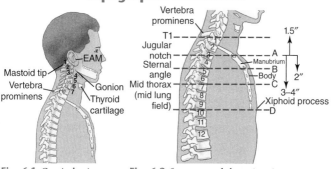

Fig. 6.1 Cervical spine landmarks.

Fig. 6.2 Sternum and thoracic spine landmarks.

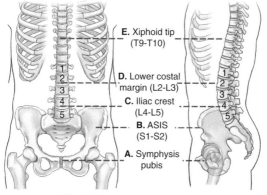

Fig. 6.3 Lower spine landmarks.

175

AP "Open Mouth" C1-C2: Cervical Spine
Atlas and Axis

Warning: For trauma patients, do not remove cervical collar and do not move their head or neck until authorized by a physician who has evaluated the horizontal beam lateral image or CT scan of the cervical spine.

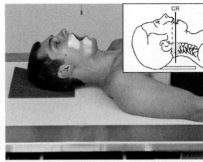

Fig. 6.4 AP open mouth for C1-C2.

- 18 × 24 cm (8 × 10") portrait
- Grid
- AEC not recommended because of small field

Position
- Supine or erect, patient centered to CR and centerline
- Adjust patient's head without opening his or her mouth—a line from lower margin of upper incisors to the base of the skull (mastoid tips) is perpendicular to table and/or IR, or angle the CR accordingly
- Center IR to CR
- As a last step before making exposure—have patient open mouth wide without moving head (make final check for head alignment)

Central Ray: CR ⊥ to IR through midportion of open mouth (to C1-C2)
SID: 40" (102 cm)
Collimation: Close collimation to C1-C2 region
Respiration: Suspend during exposure

kV Range:	Analog: **70–80 kV**			Digital Systems: **80 ± 5 kV**		
	cm	kV	mA	Time	mAs	SID	Exposure Indicator
S							
M							
L							

176   Bontrager Textbook, 9th ed, p. 310.

AP (PA) for Dens: Cervical Spine
AP (Fuchs Method) and PA (Judd Method)

Warning: Do not attempt on possible cervical trauma.
- 18 × 24 cm (8 × 10″) landscape
- Grid
- AEC not recommended

Position
- Supine or erect, MSP aligned to centerline, no rotation
- Elevate chin until MML is near ⊥ to IR (may require some cephalic CR angle if chin cannot be elevated sufficiently)

Note: May also be taken PA (Judd method) with chin against tabletop, with same CR alignment.

- Center IR to exiting CR

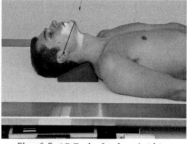

Fig. 6.5 AP Fuchs for dens (within foramen magnum outline).

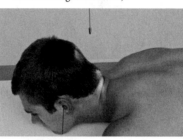

Fig. 6.6 PA Judd method.

Central Ray: CR parallel to MML; 1″ (2.5 cm) inferoposterior to mastoid tips and angles of mandible
SID: 40″ (102 cm)
Collimation: Close collimation to C1-C2 region
Respiration: Suspend during exposure

6

Vertebral Column

	cm	kV	mA	Time	mAs	SID	Exposure Indicator
S							
M							
L							

kV Range: Analog: **70–80 kV**   Digital Systems: **80 ± 5 kV**

AP "Open Mouth" and AP (PA) Dens

Evaluation Criteria
Anatomy
Demonstrated

- **Open mouth:** Dens (odontoid process) and vertebral body of C2, lateral masses and transverse processes of C1, and C1-C2 atlantoaxial joints
- **AP Fuchs:** Dens (odontoid process) within foramen magnum

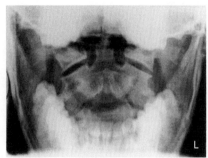

Fig. 6.7 AP open mouth—dens.

Competency Check: _____

Technologist   Date

Position

- **Open mouth:** Upper incisors and base of the skull superimposed. Entire dens demonstrated within foramen magnum
- **AP Fuchs:** Tip of mandible not superimposed over dens. Symmetric appearance of mandible

Fig. 6.8 AP (AP Fuchs—dens).

Competency Check: _____

Technologist   Date

Exposure

- Optimal density (brightness) and contrast
- Soft tissue margins, bony margins and trabecular markings. Sharp outline of dens; no motion

AP Axial: Cervical Spine

- 18 × 24 cm (8 × 10″) or 24 × 30 cm (10 × 12″) portrait
- Grid

Position

- Supine or erect, center midsagittal plane to CR (and to centerline of IR)
- Raise patient's chin slightly, as needed, so the CR angle superimposes the mentum of the mandible over the base of the skull (to prevent mandible from superimposing more than C1-C2)
- Center IR to projected CR

Central Ray: CR 15°–20° cephalad, to enter at C4 (inferior margin of thyroid cartilage)

SID: 40″ (102 cm)

Collimation: On four sides to anatomy of interest

Respiration: Suspend during exposure

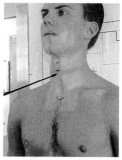

Fig. 6.9 Erect AP (CR 15°–20° cephalad).

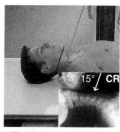

Fig. 6.10 Supine AP (CR 15°–20° cephalad).

kV Range:		Analog: 70–80 kV			Digital Systems: 80 ± 5 kV		
	cm	kV	mA	Time	mAs	SID	Exposure Indicator
S							
M							
L							

Bontrager Textbook, 9th ed, p. 311.

6

Vertebral Column

Oblique: Cervical Spine

Warning: Do not attempt if there is possible cervical trauma. Right and left obliques imaged for comparison (as either posterior or anterior obliques); **anterior obliques result in less thyroid dose**

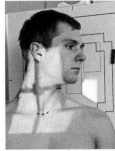

Fig. 6.11 LPO; CR 15° cephalad.

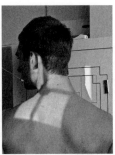

Fig. 6.12 RAO; CR 15° caudad.

- 24 × 30 cm (10 × 12″) portrait
- Grid (optional for small patient or pediatrics)

Position

- Erect preferred (sitting or standing), entire torso and head turned 45° to IR, C spine aligned to CR (and centerline of IR)
- Have patient raise chin slightly, looking straight ahead (turn head slightly toward IR to prevent superimposing C1 by ramus of mandible)
- Center IR to projected CR

Central Ray (Posterior Obliques): CR 15°–20° **cephalad**, to enter at C4. 15°–20° **caudad** angle required for anterior oblique

SID: 40–72″ (102–183 cm)—Longer SID recommended

Collimation: To C spine region

Respiration: Suspend during exposure

		cm	kV	mA	Time	mAs	SID	Exposure Indicator
kV Range:	Analog: 70–80 kV			Digital Systems: 80 ± 5 kV				
S								
M								
L								

Bontrager Textbook, 9th ed, p. 312.

6

Vertebral Column

AP Axial and Oblique: Cervical Spine

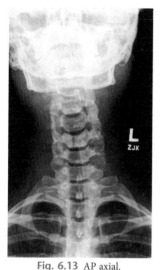

Fig. 6.13 AP axial.

Competency Check: _____

Technologist   Date

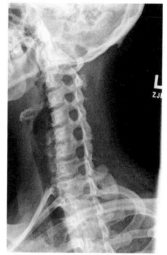

Fig. 6.14 RPO.

Competency Check: _____

Technologist   Date

Evaluation Criteria

Anatomy Demonstrated

- **AP axial:** C3–T2 vertebral bodies and intervertebral joints
- **Oblique:** Intervertebral foramina open and pedicles
- **LPO/RPO projections:** Demonstrate upside (farthest from IR) intervertebral foramina and pedicles
- **LAO/RAO projections:** Demonstrate downside (closest to IR) intervertebral foramina and pedicles

Position

- **AP axial:** Intervertebral joints open and spinous processes equidistant to midline
- **Oblique: 45° (AP or PA):** Intervertebral foramina uniformly open and pedicles in profile

Exposure

- Optimal density (brightness) and contrast; no motion
- Soft tissue and bony margins and trabecular markings sharp

Vertebral Column

Lateral (Erect): Cervical Spine

Trauma patients: See Trauma Series: Cervical Spine

- 24 × 30 cm (10 × 12″) portrait
- Grid (optional for small or pediatric patients)

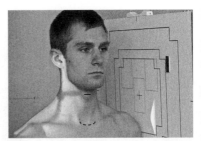

Fig. 6.15 Erect lateral, 72″ (183 cm) SID.

Position

- Erect (sitting or standing) in lateral position, C spine aligned and centered to CR (and centerline of IR)
- Top of IR ≈1–2″ (3–5 cm) above level of EAM
- Elevate patient's chin slightly (to remove mandible angles from spine)
- Relax and depress both shoulders evenly (weights in each hand may be necessary to visualize C7)

Note: See following page for swimmer's lateral if C7 is still not visualized.

Central Ray: CR ⊥ IR to level of C4 (upper thyroid cartilage)

SID: 60–72″ (153–183 cm) (Longer SID provides for better visualization of C7 because of less divergent rays)

Collimation: On four sides to C spine region

Respiration: Expose on complete expiration

kV Range:	Analog: 70–80 kV			Digital Systems: 80 ± 5 kV		

	cm	kV	mA	Time	mAs	SID	Exposure Indicator
S							
M							
L							

Bontrager Textbook, 9th ed, p. 313.

6

Vertebral Column

Cervicothoracic (Swimmer's) Lateral: Cervical Spine

C5-T3 Region

- 24 × 30 cm (10 × 12")
  portrait
- Grid

Position

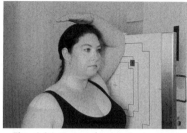

Fig. 6.16 Cervicothoracic (swimmer's) lateral.

- Erect (sitting or standing) preferred; align C spine to CR (and centerline of IR)
- Elevate arm and shoulder closest to IR, and rotate this shoulder slightly anteriorly or posteriorly
- Opposite arm down, relax and depress shoulder, with slight opposite rotation (from other shoulder) to separate humeral heads from vertebra. May also be taken in lateral recumbent position with one arm and shoulder down and one up (trauma alternative)

Central Ray: CR ⊥ centered to T1 (approximately 1" [2.5 cm] above level of jugular notch); **optional** 3°–5° caudad to separate the two shoulders for patient with limited flexibility

SID: 60–72" (153–183 cm)

Collimation: Collimate closely to area of interest

Respiration: Expose on full expiration or orthostatic (breathing) technique

kV Range:	Analog: 75–85 kV			Digital Systems: 90 ± 5 kV			
	cm	kV	mA	Time	mAs	SID	Exposure Indicator
S							
M							
L							

6

Vertebral Column

Lateral (Erect) and Cervicothoracic (Swimmer's) Lateral: Cervical Spine

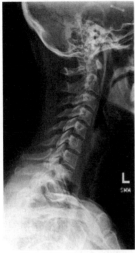
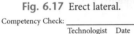

Fig. 6.17 Erect lateral.

Competency Check: _____
                   Technologist   Date

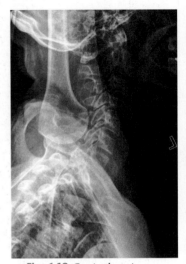

Fig. 6.18 Cervicothoracic (swimmer's) lateral.

Competency Check: _____
                   Technologist   Date

Evaluation Criteria

Anatomy Demonstrated

- **Lateral:** C1-C7 (minimum) intervertebral joint spaces and vertebral bodies demonstrated
- **Cervicothoracic:** Vertebral bodies and intervertebral disk spaces from C5-T3 (minimum) demonstrated

Position

- **Lateral:** Near superimposition of zygapophyseal joints; no superimposition of mandible on C spine
- **Cervicothoracic:** Separation of humeral heads from C spine; vertebral bodies in lateral perspective

Exposure

- Optimal density (brightness) and contrast of lower cervical and upper thoracic spine; no motion
- Soft tissue margins and bony anatomy visible

Lateral (Hyperflexion and Hyperextension): Cervical Spine

Warning: Functional study. Do **not** attempt on possible trauma patients.
- 24 × 30 cm (10 × 12″) portrait
- Grid or nongrid

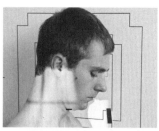

Fig. 6.19 Hyperflexion.

Position
- Erect preferred (sitting or standing) in true lateral position, C spine aligned to CR (and centerline of IR)
- Relax and depress shoulders as much as possible

First IR: Depress chin to touch chest, if possible

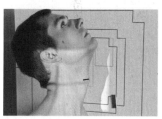

Fig. 6.20 Hyperextension.

Second IR: Elevate chin as far as is comfortable (entire C spine is included on both projections)

Central Ray: **CR** ⊥ to C4 (level of upper margin of thyroid cartilage)

SID: 60–72″ (153–183 cm)

Collimation: To C spine area

Respiration: Expose on full expiration

---

kV Range:	Analog: 70–80 kV				Digital Systems: 80 ± 5 kV	
	cm	kV	mA	Time	mAs	SID	Exposure Indicator
S							
M							
L							

Vertebral Column   6

Lateral (Hyperflexion and Hyperextension): Cervical Spine

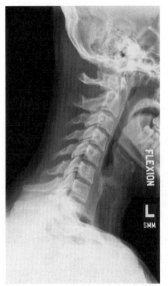

Fig. 6.21 Hyperflexion lateral.

Competency Check: _____
                     Technologist   Date

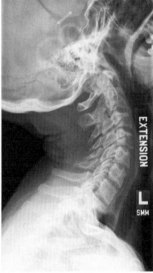

Fig. 6.22 Hyperextension lateral.

Competency Check: _____
                     Technologist   Date

Evaluation Criteria

Anatomy Demonstrated

- **C1-C7:** Range of motion and ligament stability demonstrated

Position

- **Hyperflexion:** Spinous processes well separated
- **Hyperextension:** Spinous processes in close proximity

Exposure

- Optimal density (brightness) and contrast; no motion
- Soft tissue margins visible and trabecular markings sharp

Trauma Series: Cervical Spine

Warning: Do not remove cervical collar unless so indicated by the physician after viewing horizontal beam lateral.

Horizontal Beam Lateral
- 24 × 30 cm (10 × 12″) portrait
- Grid or nongrid
- **SID:** 60–72″ (153–183 cm)
- CR ⊥ to C4 (upper thyroid cartilage) (top of IR ≈3–5 cm or 1–2″ above EAM)

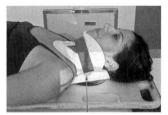

Fig. 6.23 Horizontal beam lateral.

AP
- Depress shoulders
- 24 × 30 cm (10 × 12″) portrait
- Grid
- **SID:** 40–48″ (102–123 cm)
- **CR:** 15°–20° cephalad, to enter at C4
- Expose upon full expiration

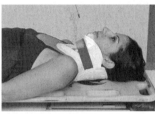

Fig. 6.24 AP axial.

AP Axial Oblique
- 24 × 30 cm (10 × 12″) portrait
- Grid
- **SID:** 40–48″ (102–123 cm)
- **CR:** 45° medially (and 15° cephalad if nongrid)
- CR to enter at level of C4

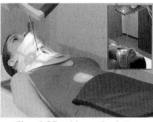

Fig. 6.25 Oblique (both R and L obliques).

Cervicothoracic Lateral
(Optional projection if needed to visualize C7)
- 24 × 30 cm (10 × 12″) portrait
- Grid
- Elevate shoulder and arm nearest IR. Depress opposite shoulder
- **SID:** 40–48″ (102–123 cm)
- **CR:** IR centered to T1 (approximately 1.5″ [2.5 cm] above level of jugular notch)

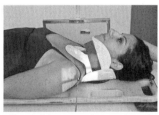

Fig. 6.26 Cervicothoracic lateral.

6

Vertebral Column

AP: Thoracic Spine

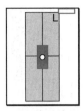

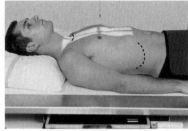

Fig. 6.27 AP thoracic spine.

- 35 × 43 cm (14 × 17″) portrait
- Grid
- Lower thoracolumbar spine at cathode end (anode heel effect)
- Wedge compensation filter recommended to produce uniform density of spine recommended

Position

- Supine, spine aligned and centered to midline of table and/or IR; flex hips and knees to reduce lordotic curvature
- Ensure top of IR is at least 1½″ (3 cm) above shoulder
- Ensure no rotation of thorax or pelvis; shield radiosensitive tissues

Central Ray: CR ⊥ to center of IR (at level of T7 [as for an AP chest], 3–4″ or 8–10 cm below jugular notch)

SID: 40″ (102 cm)

Collimation: Long narrow collimation field to T spine region

Respiration: Expose on expiration for more uniform density

kV Range:		Analog: 75–85 kV			Digital Systems: 85 ± 5 kV	

	cm	kV	mA	Time	mAs	SID	Exposure Indicator
S							
M							
L							

Bontrager Textbook, 9th ed, p. 320.

Lateral: Thoracic Spine

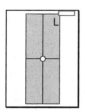

- 35 × 43 cm (14 × 17″) portrait
- Grid
- Lead mat placed on table posterior to patient to reduce scatter
- Do not use AEC if orthostatic breathing technique is used

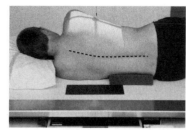

Fig. 6.28 Lateral thoracic spine.

Position

- Recumbent, support under head, lateral with knees flexed, arms raised, and elbows flexed. Shield radiosensitive tissues
- Align and center midaxillary plane to midline of table and/or IR
- Ensure top of IR is at least 1½″ (3 cm) above shoulders; no rotation
- Supports should be placed under lower back, as needed, to straighten and align spine near parallel to tabletop (A slight natural curvature corresponding to divergent rays is helpful)

Central Ray: CR ⊥ to center of IR T7 (3–4″ [8–10 cm] below jugular notch or 7–8″ [18–21 cm] below the vertebra prominens). A patient with broad shoulders may require a 10°–15° cephalic CR angle if waist is not supported

SID: 40″ (102 cm)

Collimation: Long, narrow collimation field to T spine region

Respiration: Orthostatic (breathing) technique recommended—minimum of 2–3 seconds; or expose on full inspiration

kV Range:	Analog: 80–90 kV		Digital Systems: 90 ± 5 kV			

	cm	kV	mA	Time	mAs	SID	Exposure Indicator
S							
M							
L							

6

Vertebral Column

AP and Lateral: Thoracic Spine

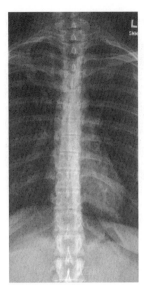

Fig. 6.29 AP thoracic spine.

Competency Check: _____
                   Technologist Date

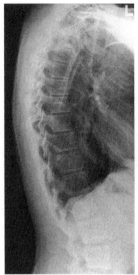

Fig. 6.30 Lateral thoracic spine (suspended respiration).

Competency Check: _____
                   Technologist Date

Evaluation Criteria

Anatomy Demonstrated
- **AP and lateral:** 12 thoracic bodies, intervertebral joint spaces, and spinous and transverse processes

Position
- **AP:** SC joints equidistant from midline, no rotation
- **Lateral:** Intervertebral disk spaces open

Exposure
- Optimal density (brightness) and contrast; no motion on AP projection. Breathing technique for lateral projection is desirable
- Soft tissue margins visible and trabecular markings sharp

190

6

Vertebral Column

Oblique: Thoracic Spine

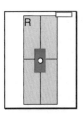

Both oblique projections generally imaged for comparison. May also take as anterior oblique (lower breast dose)
- 35 × 43 cm (14 × 17″) portrait
- Grid

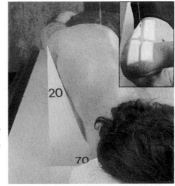

Fig. 6.31 70° RPO (20° from lateral).

Position
- Recumbent or erect, rotated posteriorly 20° from true lateral
- Align and center spine to midline of table and/or IR; place arm away from IR behind back and arm closest to IR up in front of head
- Ensure top of IR is at least 1½″ (3 cm) above shoulders

Central Ray: CR ⊥ to center of IR to T7 (3–4″ [8–10 cm] below jugular notch or 2″ [5 cm] below sternal angle)

SID: 40″ (102 cm)

Collimation: Long, narrow collimation field to T spine region

Respiration: Expose on expiration

kV Range:		Analog: 75–85 kV		Digital Systems: 90 ± 5 kV		
	cm	kV	mA	Time	mAs	SID	Exposure Indicator
S							
M							
L							

Vertebral Column

6

AP (PA): Lumbar Spine

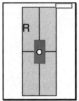

Note: May be taken PA for better opening of intervertebral spaces by divergent rays.

- 30 × 35 cm (11 × 14″) portrait or 35 × 43 cm (14 × 17″) portrait
- Grid

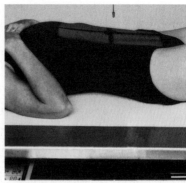

Fig. 6.32 AP lumbar, hips and knees flexed.

Position (AP)

- Supine, spine aligned to midline of table and/or grid
- Flex hips and knees (to reduce lordotic curvature)
- No rotation (ASISs same distance from table)
- Center IR to CR

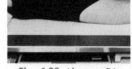

Fig. 6.33 Alternate PA.

Central Ray: CR ⊥ to ≈1½″ (4 cm) above iliac crest (L3); or center at crest for 35 × 43 cm IR

SID: 40″ (102 cm)

Collimation: Long, narrow collimation field to L spine region (include SI joints)

Respiration: Expose at end of expiration

kV Range:	Analog: 75–85 kV			Digital Systems: 85 ± 5 kV			
	cm	kV	mA	Time	mAs	SID	Exposure Indicator
S							
M							
L							

Bontrager Textbook, 9th ed, p. 337.

Vertebral Column

6

AP (PA): Lumbar Spine

Evaluation Criteria

Anatomy Demonstrated
- T12-S1 (minimum) demonstrated
- Lumbar vertebral bodies, intervertebral joints, spinous and transverse processes, SI joints and sacrum

Position
- No rotation evident by symmetry of transverse processes, SI joints, and sacrum
- Spinous processes are midline

Exposure
- Optimal density (brightness) and contrast; no motion
- Soft tissue margins and sharp trabecular markings clearly demonstrated

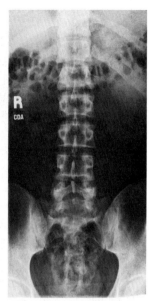

Fig. 6.34 AP lumbar spine.

Competency Check: _____

Technologist   Date

6

Vertebral Column

Lateral: Lumbar Spine

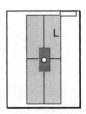

- 30 × 35 cm (11 × 14″) portrait or 35 × 43 cm (14 × 17″) portrait
- Grid
- Lower lumbar spine at cathode end
- Lead masking posterior to patient

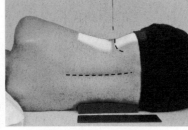

Fig. 6.35 Lateral L spine.

Position

- Recumbent in true lateral position, flex hips and knees, align and center midaxillary plane to centerline
- Place support under waist, as needed, to place entire spine parallel to tabletop (see *Note*). Provide support between knees
- Center IR to CR

Central Ray: CR ⊥ to level of ≈1½″ (4 cm) above iliac crest (L3), or at iliac crest (L4) for 35 × 43 cm (14 × 17″) IR

SID: 40″ (102 cm)

Collimation: Long, narrow collimation field to L spine region

Respiration: Expose at end of expiration

Note: Patient with wide pelvis and narrow thorax may require a 3°–5° caudal CR angle, even with support under waist. If patient has natural lateral curvature (scoliosis), place "sag" or convexity down.

kV Range:	Analog: 80–90 kV	Digital Systems: 85 ± 5 kV

	cm	kV	mA	Time	mAs	SID	Exposure Indicator
S							
M							
L							

Bontrager Textbook, 9th ed, p. 339.

Lateral L5-S1: Lumbar Spine

- 18 × 24 cm (8 × 10″) portrait
- Grid
- Lead masking posterior to patient

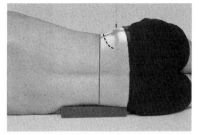

Fig. 6.36 Lateral L5-S1.

Position

- Recumbent in true lateral position, flex hips and knees, midaxillary plane aligned to midline of table and/or IR and CR
- Place support under waist, as needed, to place entire spine parallel to tabletop. Provide support between knees
- Center IR to CR

Central Ray:

- CR ⊥ to IR if entire spine is parallel to table; or 5°–8° caudad if entire spine is not parallel (most often on females). Angle CR to be parallel to the **interiliac plane**
- CR to 1.5″ (4 cm) inferior to iliac crest and 2″ (5 cm) posterior to ASIS

SID: 40″ (102 cm)

Collimation: Collimate closely to area of interest

Respiration: Suspend during exposure

	cm	kV	mA	Time	mAs	SID	Exposure Indicator
S							
M							
L							

kV Range: Analog: 85–95 kV Digital Systems: 90 ± 5 kV

6

Vertebral Column

Lateral and Lateral L5-S1: Lumbar Spine

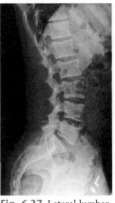

Fig. 6.37 Lateral lumbar spine.

Competency Check: _____

Technologist   Date

Fig. 6.38 Lateral L5-S1.

Competency Check: _____

Technologist   Date

Evaluation Criteria

Anatomy Demonstrated

- **Lateral:** L1-L4 vertebral bodies, intervertebral joints, and foramina and spinous processes
- **Lateral L5-S1:** Open L5-S1 vertebral bodies, intervertebral joint spaces, and intervertebral foramina

Position

- **Lateral:** Vertebral column parallel to IR; intervertebral joint spaces and foramina open; no rotation
- **Lateral L5-S1:** Intervertebral joint spaces and intervertebral foramina open; no rotation

Exposure

- Optimal density (brightness) and contrast; no motion
- Soft tissue margins visible and bony detail of vertebral bodies, joint spaces, and spinous process

Oblique: Lumbar Spine

Both oblique projections generally imaged for comparison (as either anterior or posterior obliques).

- 30 × 35 cm (11 × 14") portrait or 24 × 30 cm (10 × 12") portrait
- Grid

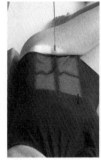

Fig. 6.39 Posterior oblique (45° RPO).

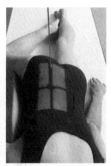

Fig. 6.40 Anterior oblique (45° LAO).

Position

- Rotate body 45° and right and left posterior or anterior obliques (use support angle blocks under pelvis and shoulders to maintain position for posterior obliques)
- Align and center spine to CR and midline of table and/or IR

Central Ray: CR ⊥ to body of L3 at level of lower costal margin (1–2" [2.5–5 cm] above iliac crest) and 2" (5 cm) medial to upside ASIS

SID: 40" (102 cm)

Collimation: To area of interest

Respiration: Suspend during exposure

Note: 50° oblique is best for L1-L2 zygapophyseal joints, and 30° for L5-S1

kV Range:		Analog: 75–85 kV			Digital Systems: 85 ± 5 kV		
	cm	kV	mA	Time	mAs	SID	Exposure Indicator
S							
M							
L							

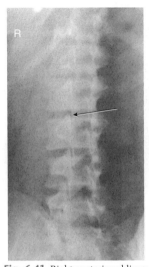

Fig. 6.41 Right posterior oblique.

Competency Check: _____
Technologist   Date

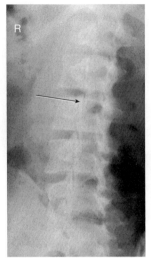

Fig. 6.42 Right anterior oblique.

Competency Check: _____
Technologist   Date

Evaluation Criteria

Anatomy Demonstrated

- **LPO/RPO:** L1-L4 downside zygapophyseal joints. Scottie dog elements visible
- **LAO/RAO:** L1-L4 upside zygapophyseal joints. Scottie dog elements visible

Position

- Zygapophyseal joints and pedicle ("eye") centered on the vertebral body

Exposure

- Optimal density (brightness) and contrast; no motion
- Soft tissue margins visible and bony detail of vertebral bodies, joint spaces, and elements of Scottie dog (arrows indicate zygapophyseal joints)

6

Vertebral Column

198

PA: Scoliosis Series
Ferguson Method

PA greatly reduces dose to radiation-sensitive areas and is highly recommended over AP projection.

A scoliosis series frequently includes two PA (or AP) images taken for comparison, one erect and one recumbent.

- 35 × 43 cm (14 × 17″) portrait or 35 × 90 cm (14 × 36″) portrait
- Grid
- Compensating filters to produce a more uniform density of spine

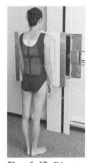

Fig. 6.43 PA without block.

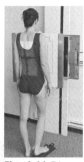

Fig. 6.44 PA with block under foot on convex side of curve.

Position

First IR:

- Erect, standing or seated, spine aligned and centered to midline of table and/or IR, arms at side, no rotation of pelvis or thorax
- Lower margin of IR 1–2″ (2.5–5 cm) below iliac crest

Second IR: Place 3- to 4-inch (8- to 10-cm) block under foot (or buttock if seated) on **convex side** of curvature (Identifies primary deforming curves from compensatory curve)

Shielding: Use gonad and breast shields

Central Ray: CR ⊥ to center of IR

SID: 40–60″ (102–153 cm); longer SID is recommended

Collimation: Long and narrow to vertebral column region

Respiration: On full expiration

kV Range:	Analog: 80–90 kV			Digital Systems: 85 ± 5 kV		
	cm	kV	mA	Time	mAs	SID	Exposure Indicator
S							
M							
L							

Bontrager Textbook, 9th ed., p. 344.

6

Vertebral Column

AP: Lumbar Spine
Right and Left Bending

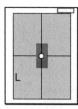

Note: May be taken erect PA to reduce dose to radiation-sensitive areas.

- 35 × 43 cm (14 × 17″) portrait or 35 × 90 cm (14 × 36″) portrait
- Grid
- Compensating filters to produce a more uniform density of spine

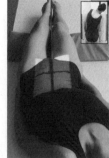

Fig. 6.45 AP, right bending.

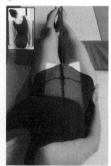

Fig. 6.46 AP, left bending.

Position
- Supine or erect, spine centered to CR and midline of table and/or IR
- Bend laterally as far as possible (right then left) without tilting pelvis (pelvis remains stationary and acts as a fulcrum)
- Ensure no rotation of pelvis and upper torso
- Lower margin of IR 1–2″ (2.5–5 cm) below iliac crest

Central Ray: CR ⊥ to center of IR (higher centering if thoracic spine is area of interest)

SID: 40–60″ (102–153 cm)

Collimation: Include vertebral column of interest

Respiration: Expose at end of expiration

kV Range:	Analog: 80–90 kV			Digital Systems: 85 ± 5 kV		
	cm	kV	mA	Time	mAs	SID	Exposure Indicator
S							
M							
L							

Bontrager Textbook, 9th ed, p. 345.

Lateral (Hyperflexion and Hyperextension): Lumbar Spine

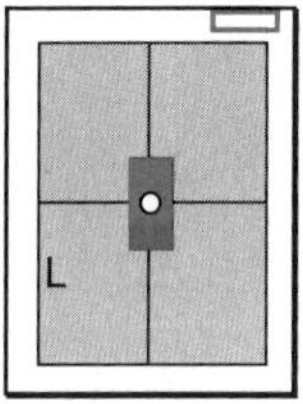

- 35 × 43 cm (14 × 17″) portrait
- Grid
- Lead masking posterior to patient

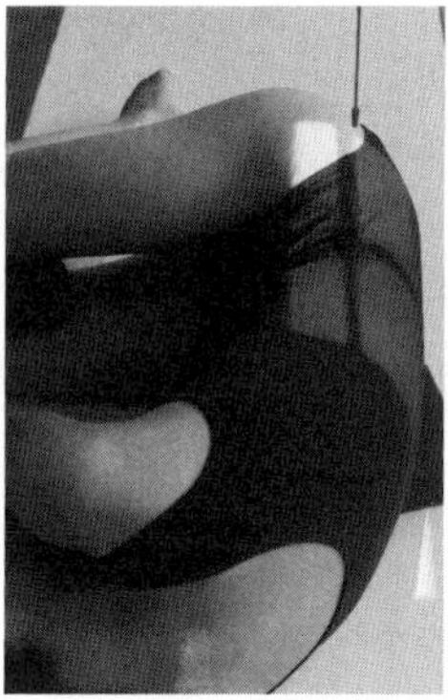

Fig. 6.47 Hyperflexion lateral.

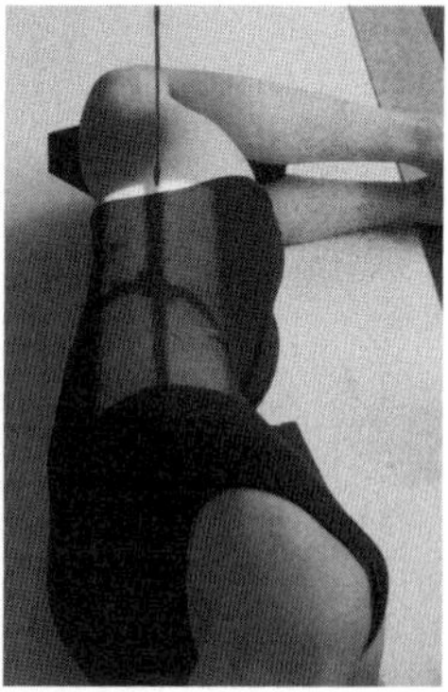

Fig. 6.48 Hyperextension lateral.

Position

- Recumbent or erect, spine centered to table
- Support under waist to align spine parallel to tabletop
- Hyperflex forward as far as possible, then hyperextend back as far as possible for second IR; maintain true lateral position
- Lower margin of IR 1–2″ (2.5–5 cm) below iliac crest

Central Ray: CR ⊥ to center of IR (or to site of fusion if known)
SID: 40″ (102 cm)
Collimation: On four sides to near borders of IR
Respiration: Expose at end of expiration

kV Range: Analog: 85–95 kV Digital Systems: 90 ± 5 kV

	cm	kV	mA	Time	mAs	SID	Exposure Indicator
S							
M							
L							

Bontrager Textbook, 9th ed, p. 346.

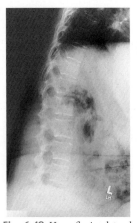

Fig. 6.49 Hyperflexion lateral.

Competency Check: _____

Technologist   Date

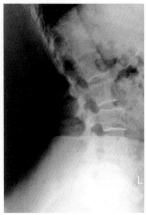

Fig. 6.50 Hyperextension lateral.

Competency Check: _____

Technologist   Date

Evaluation Criteria

Anatomy Demonstrated

- **Hyperflexion:** Thoracic and lumbar vertebra including 1–2″ (≈3–5 cm) of the iliac crests. Lateral view of lumbar vertebrae in hyperflexion
- **Hyperextension:** Thoracic and lumbar vertebra including 1–2″ (≈3–5 cm) of the iliac crests. Lateral view of lumbar vertebrae in hyperextension

Position

- **Hyperflexion:** True lateral with no rotation; spaces between spinous processes open
- **Hyperextension:** True lateral with no rotation; spaces between spinous processes closed

Exposure

- Optimal density (brightness) and contrast; no motion
- Bony detail of vertebral bodies, spinous processes, and intervertebral joint spaces

202

AP Axial: Sacrum

- 24 × 30 cm (10 × 12″) portrait
- Grid

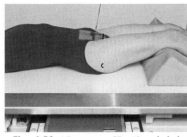

Fig. 6.51 AP sacrum, CR 15° cephalad.

Position
- Supine, spine centered to CR and midline of table and/or IR
- No rotation of pelvis (both ASIS same distance from table)
- Center IR to projected CR (Shield radiosensitive tissues. Shield gonads for males.)

Central Ray: CR 15° cephalad, at 2″ (5 cm) superior to pubic symphysis

SID: 40″ (102 cm)

Collimation: On four sides to area of sacrum

Respiration: Suspend during exposure

6

Vertebral Column

kV Range: Analog: 75–80 kV   Digital Systems: 85 ± 5 kV

	cm	kV	mA	Time	mAs	SID	Exposure Indicator
S							
M							
L							

AP Axial: Coccyx

Note: May be done PA with 10°
cephalic angle if patient cannot
sustain weight on the coccyx
area in a supine position.
Urinary bladder should be
emptied before procedure is
performed.

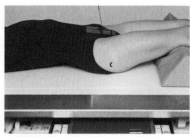

Fig. 6.52 AP axial coccyx, CR 10°
caudad.

- 18 × 24 cm (8 × 10″) portrait
- Grid
- Cautious use of AEC

Position
- Supine, support under knees, shield radiosensitive tissue, gonad
  shield for males
- Align and center midsagittal plane to midline of table and/or IR,
  no rotation
- Center IR to level of projected CR

Central Ray: CR 10° caudad, centered to 2″ (5 cm) superior to
symphysis pubis

SID: 40″ (102 cm)

Collimation: Close collimation to area of coccyx

Respiration: Suspend during exposure

kV Range:		Analog: 75–80 kV		Digital Systems: 80 ± 5 kV		
	cm	kV	mA	Time	mAs	SID	Exposure Indicator
S							
M							
L							

Bontrager Textbook, 9th ed, p. 348.

AP Axial: Sacrum and Coccyx

Evaluation Criteria

Anatomy Demonstrated

- **AP sacrum:** Nonforeshortened image of sacrum
- **AP coccyx:** Nonforeshortened image of coccyx

Position

- **AP sacrum:** Sacrum free of superimposition and sacral foramina visible
- **AP coccyx:** Coccyx free of superimposition and not rotated

Exposure

- Optimal density (brightness) and contrast; no motion
- Soft tissue visible and sharp bony detail

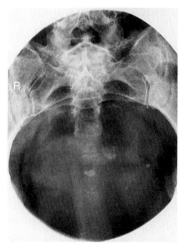

Fig. 6.53 AP axial sacrum.

Competency Check: _____
Technologist   Date

Fig. 6.54 AP axial coccyx.

Competency Check: _____
Technologist   Date

6

Vertebral Column

Lateral: Sacrum and Coccyx

Note: Lateral sacrum and lateral coccyx may be taken as one projection if both sacrum and coccyx are being examined (reduces patient exposure).

- 24 × 30 cm (10 × 12″) portrait
- Grid
- Lead masking posterior to patient
- Use of boomerang-type compensating filter is recommended if coccyx is to be included

Position

- Lateral recumbent, hips and knees flexed, true lateral position
- Center sacrum to CR and midline of table and/or IR (Align patient and IR to correctly centered CR)

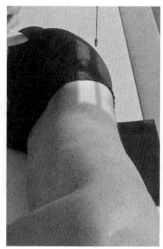

Fig. 6.55 Lateral sacrum and coccyx.

Central Ray (Sacrum): CR ⊥, directed to 3–4″ (8–10 cm) posterior to upside ASIS

SID: 40″ (102 cm)

Collimation: On four sides to area of sacrum

Respiration: Suspend during exposure

	cm	kV	mA	Time	mAs	SID	Exposure Indicator
kV Range:		Analog: 85–95 kV			Digital Systems: 90 ± 5 kV		
S							
M							
L							

Bontrager Textbook, 9th ed., p. 349.

6

Vertebral Column

Lateral: Coccyx

Note: Lateral sacrum and lateral coccyx are commonly taken as one projection if both sacrum and coccyx are being examined (reduces patient exposure).
- 18 × 24 cm (8 × 10") portrait
- Grid
- Lead masking posterior to patient
- Cautious use of AEC

Position
- Lateral recumbent, with hips and knees flexed 90°, true lateral position

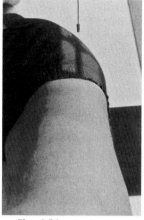

Fig. 6.56 Lateral coccyx.

- Center coccyx to CR and midline of table and/or IR (remember the coccyx is located superficially between buttocks slightly superior to level of greater trochanter)
- Center IR to CR

Central Ray: CR ⊥ to 2" (5 cm) distal to level of ASIS and 3–4" (8–10 cm) posterior

SID: 40" (102 cm)

Collimation: To area of distal sacrum and coccyx

Respiration: Suspend during exposure

---

kV Range:		Analog: 75–85 kV		Digital Systems: 85 ± 5 kV		
	cm	kV	mA	Time	mAs	SID	Exposure Indicator
S							
M							
L							

6

Vertebral Column

Evaluation Criteria
Anatomy Demonstrated

- Lateral view of sacrum and coccyx
- Lateral view of L5-S1 intervertebral joint

Position

- No rotation evident by greater sciatic notches and femoral heads superimposed
- Entire sacrum and coccyx included

Exposure

- Optimal density (brightness) and contrast; no motion
- Trabecular markings clearly demonstrated

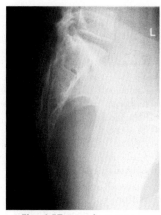

Fig. 6.57 Lateral sacrum and coccyx.

Competency Check: _____
Technologist   Date

AP Axial: Sacroiliac (SI) Joint

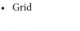

- 24 × 30 cm (10 × 12″) portrait
- Grid

Position

- Supine, center patient to midline of table and/or IR

Fig. 6.58 AP axial SI joints (CR 30°–35° cephalad).

- No rotation of pelvis (ASISs the same distance from tabletop)
- Center IR to projected CR. Shield radiosensitive tissues **as well as gonads** for males

Central Ray: CR 30° (males) and 35° (females) cephalad, 2″ (5 cm) below level of ASIS

SID: 40″ (102 cm)

Collimation: Four sides to area of interest

Respiration: Suspend during exposure

Vertebral Column

	cm	kV	mA	Time	mAs	SID	Exposure Indicator
S							
M							
L							

kV Range: Analog: 80–90 kV   Digital Systems: 85 ± 5 kV

Posterior Oblique: Sacroiliac (SI) Joint

- 24 × 30 cm (10 × 12″) portrait
- Grid
- Bilateral for comparison

Position

- Patient in 25°–30° posterior oblique with side of interest elevated (use support to maintain this position)
- Align elevated SI joint to CR and to midline of table and/ or IR (1″ [2.5 cm] medial to upside ASIS)
- Center IR to CR

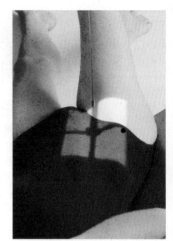

Fig. 6.59 25°–30° LPO for upside (right) SI joint.

- Shield radiosensitive tissue **as well as gonads** for males

Central Ray: CR ⊥ to 1″ (2.5 cm) medial to elevated ASIS

SID: 40″ (102 cm)

Collimation: Four sides to area of interest

Respiration: Suspend during exposure

Note: CR may be angled 15°–20° cephalad to best demonstrate the distal part of joint

	cm	kV	mA	Time	mAs	SID	Exposure Indicator
kV Range:		Analog: 80–90 kV			Digital Systems: 85 ± 5 kV		
S							
M							
L							

Bontrager Textbook, 9th ed, p. 352.

6

Vertebral Column

Posterior Oblique: Sacroiliac Joint

Evaluation Criteria

Anatomy Demonstrated
- Open upside (farthest from IR) SI joint

Position
- **LPO:** Right SI joint open; no overlap of iliac wing and sacrum
- **RPO:** Left SI joint open; no overlap of iliac wing and sacrum

Exposure
- Optimal density (brightness) and contrast; no motion
- Bony margins and sharp trabecular markings clearly demonstrated

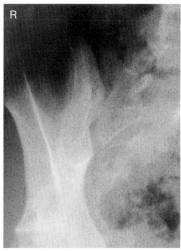

Fig. 6.60 LPO projection of (right) SI joint.

Competency Check: _____

Technologist   Date

6

Vertebral Column

Chapter 7

Bony Thorax

(R) Routine, (S) Special

Positioning Considerations
Sternum

The routine for a sternum generally includes a lateral and an oblique wherein the sternum is shifted to the left of the spine and is superimposed over the homogeneous heart shadow. A 15°–20° RAO achieves this best. An orthostatic-breathing technique generally is used to blur out the lung markings and the ribs overlying the sternum. If preferred, exposure can also be made on suspended expiration. A minimum SID for sternum radiography is 40″ (102 cm). The patient's skin should be at least 38 cm (15″) below the surface of the collimator to reduce skin dose.

Ribs

Each technologist should determine the preferred routine for his or her department.

Two-Image Routine

One suggested two-image routine is an **AP** or **PA** with the area of interest closest to the image receptor (IR) (above or below diaphragm) and an **oblique** projection of the axillary ribs on the side of injury. Therefore the oblique for this routine on an injury to the left anterior ribs would be an RAO, shifting the spine away from the area of injury and to increase visibility of the left axillary ribs. The oblique for an injury to the right posterior ribs would be an RPO wherein the spine again is rotated away from the area of injury.

Three-Image Routine

Another three-image routine required in some departments for all rib trauma consists of **AP above diaphragm** or **AP below diaphragm** and **RPO** and **LPO** of the site of injury.

Above and Below Diaphragm

The location of the injury site in relationship to the diaphragm is important for all routines. Those injuries above the diaphragm require less exposure (nearer to a chest technique) when taken on **inspiration** and those below the diaphragm require an exposure nearer to that of an abdomen technique when taken on **expiration**.

Right Anterior Oblique (RAO): Sternum

- 24 × 30 cm (10 × 12″) portrait
- Grid
- Orthostatic-breathing technique (3–4 seconds) or suspended expiration
- AEC not recommended

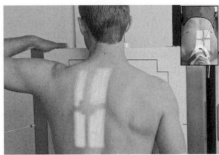

Fig. 7.1 Erect 15°–20° RAO sternum (*inset:* trauma option).

Position

- Erect (preferred) or semiprone, turned 15°–20° with right side down (RAO) (A thin-chested patient requires slightly more obliquity than a thick-chested patient)
- Center sternum to CR at midline of table or IR holder

Central Ray: CR ⊥ to midsternum (1″ [2.5 cm] to left of midline and midway between jugular notch and xiphoid process)

SID: 40″ (102 cm)

Collimation: Long, narrow collimation field to region of sternum

7

	cm	kV	mA	Time	mAs	SID	Exposure Indicator
kV Range:	Analog: 70–80 kV				Digital Systems: 80 ± 5 kV		
S							
M							
L							

Bontrager Textbook, 9th ed, p. 364.

Lateral: Sternum

- 24 × 30 cm (10 × 12″) or 35 × 35 cm (14 × 14″) portrait
- Grid
- AEC not recommended
- Place lead blocker anterior to sternum (for recumbent position)

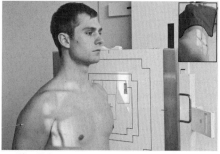

Fig. 7.2 Lateral, erect sternum (*insert:* trauma option).

Position

- Erect (preferred) (seated or standing), or lateral recumbent lying on side with vertical CR; or supine with cross-table CR for severe trauma
- Arms up above head and shoulders back
- Align sternum to CR at midline of grid or table/upright bucky
- Top of IR 1.5″ (4 cm) superior to level of jugular notch

Central Ray: CR ⊥ to midsternum

SID: 60–72″ (152–183 cm) 40″ (102 cm) minimum

Collimation: Long, narrow collimation field to region of sternum

Respiration: Expose upon **full inspiration**

kV Range:		Analog: 70–80 kV			Digital Systems: 80 ± 5 kV	
	cm	kV	mA	Time	mAs	SID	Exposure Indicator
S							
M							
L							

Oblique (RAO): Sternum

Evaluation Criteria
Anatomy Demonstrated
- Entire sternum superimposed on heart shadow

Position
- Correct patient rotation, sternum visualized alongside vertebral column

Exposure
- 3- to 4-second exposure using breathing technique; lung markings appear blurred
- Optimal contrast and density (brightness) to visualize entire sternum
- Bony margins sharp

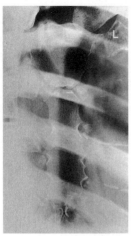

Fig. 7.3 RAO sternum.

Competency Check: _____
Technologist   Date

Lateral: Sternum

Evaluation Criteria
Anatomy Demonstrated
- Entire sternum

Position
- No rotation, sternum visualized with no superimposition on the ribs
- Shoulders and arms drawn back

Exposure
- No motion, sharp bony margins
- Optimal contrast and density (brightness) to visualize entire sternum

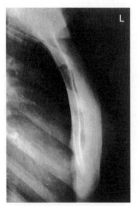

Fig. 7.4 Lateral sternum.

Competency Check: _____
Technologist   Date

Bony Thorax

7

PA and Anterior Oblique:
Sternoclavicular (SC) Joints

- 18 × 24 cm (8 × 10″) landscape
- Grid

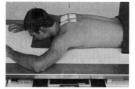

Fig. 7.5 Bilateral PA.

Position

PA: Prone or erect, midsagittal plane to center-line of CR

- Turn head to side, no rotation of shoulders
- Center **IR** to **CR**

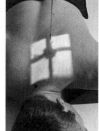

Fig. 7.6 RAO, 10°–15° oblique, CR ⊥ (both obliques commonly taken for comparison).

Oblique: Rotate thorax 10°–15° to shift vertebrae away from sternum (best visualizes **downside** SC joint). **RAO** will demonstrate the right SC joint. **LAO** will demonstrate the left SC joint.

Less obliquity (5°–10°) will best visualize the upside SC joint next to spine.

Central Ray

- **PA:** Level of T2-T3. CR ⊥ to MSP and ≈3″ (7 cm) distal to vertebra prominens (3 cm or 1.5″ inferior to jugular notch)
- **Oblique:** Level of T2-T3. CR ⊥ to 1–2″ (2.5–5 cm) lateral to MSP (toward elevated side) and ≈3″ (7 cm) distal to vertebra prominens

SID: 40″ (102 cm)

Collimation: To region of sternoclavicular joints with four-sided collimation

Respiration: Suspend respiration upon expiration

kV Range:	Analog: **70–80 kV**	Digital Systems: **80 ± 5 kV**

	cm	kV	mA	Time	mAs	SID	Exposure Indicator
S							
M							
L							

Bony Thorax

7

PA: SC Joints

Evaluation Criteria
Anatomy Demonstrated
- Lateral aspect of manubrium and medial portion of clavicles visualized lateral to vertebral column

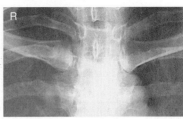

Fig. 7.7 PA bilateral SC joints.

Competency Check: _____
Technologist   Date

Position
- No rotation, equal distance of SC joints from vertebral column

Exposure
- No motion, sharp bony margins
- SC joints visualized through ribs and lungs
- Optimal contrast and density (brightness) to visualize SC joints

---

Anterior Oblique: SC Joints

Evaluation Criteria
Anatomy Demonstrated
- Manubrium and medial clavicles and downside SC joints are visualized

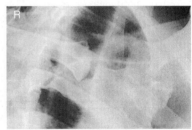

Fig. 7.8 10°–15° RAO.

Competency Check: _____
Technologist   Date

Position
- Patient rotated 10°–15°, correct rotation best demonstrates downside SC joint with no superimposition of vertebral column

Exposure
- No motion, sharp bony margins
- Contrast and density (brightness) sufficient to visualize SC joint through ribs and lungs

218

AP (or PA): Ribs (Bilateral)
Above Diaphragm

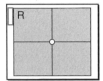

Generally taken as AP for posterior ribs and PA for anterior ribs.

- 35 × 43 cm (14 × 17″) landscape (or portrait for unilateral study or narrow chest dimensions)
- Grid

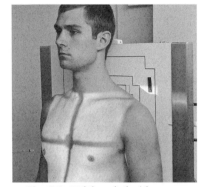

Fig. 7.9 AP bilateral ribs (above diaphragm).

Position

- Erect (preferred), or recumbent, midsagittal plane to midline of table/upright bucky and CR
- Top of IR ≈1.5″ (4 cm) above shoulders
- Roll shoulders forward, no rotation
- Ensure that thorax is centered to IR (bilateral study)

Central Ray: CR ⊥ to center of IR and 3 or 4″ (8–10 cm) below jugular notch (level of T7)

SID: 72″ (183 cm) erect; 40–48″ (102–123 cm) recumbent

Collimation: Collimate to region of interest

Respiration: Expose on **inspiration** (diaphragm down)

kV Range:		Analog: 70–80 kV		Digital Systems: 80 ± 5 kV		
	cm	kV	mA	Time	mAs	SID	Exposure Indicator
S							
M							
L							

AP: Ribs (Bilateral)
Below Diaphragm

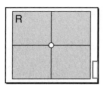

- 35 × 43 cm (14 × 17″) landscape (or portrait for unilateral study or narrow chest dimensions)
- Grid

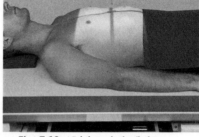

Fig. 7.10 AP bilateral ribs (below diaphragm).

Position
- Erect (preferred), or recumbent, MSP to midline of table/upright bucky and IR (and CR)
- Inferior margin of IR at iliac crest
- Ensure that both lateral margins of thorax are included (bilateral study)
- **Shield radiosensitive tissues**

Note: Some routines include only unilateral ribs of affected side.

Central Ray: CR ⊥ centered to IR at a level midway between the xiphoid process and the lower rib margin

SID: 72″ (183 cm) erect; 40″ (102 cm) recumbent

Collimation: Collimate to region of interest

Respiration: Expose on **expiration** (diaphragm at highest point)

kV Range:		Analog: 70–80 kV			Digital Systems: 80 ± 5 kV		
	cm	kV	mA	Time	mAs	SID	Exposure Indicator
S							
M							
L							

7

AP (or PA): Ribs (Bilateral)
Above and Below Diaphragm

Evaluation Criteria

Anatomy Demonstrated

Above Diaphragm
- Ribs 1–10 visualized

Below Diaphragm
- Ribs 10–12 visualized

Position
- No rotation, lateral rib margins equal distance from vertebral column

Exposure
- No motion, sharp bony margins
- Contrast and density (brightness) appropriate to visualize ribs 1–10 above diaphragm and 10–12 (minimum) below diaphragm

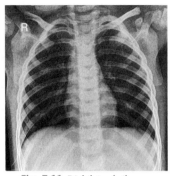

Fig. 7.11 PA bilateral ribs above diaphragm.

Competency Check: _____
Technologist   Date

Fig. 7.12 AP bilateral ribs below diaphragm.

Competency Check: _____
Technologist   Date

Anterior Oblique (RAO): Upper Axillary Ribs

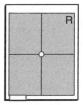

- 35 × 43 cm (14 × 17″) or 35 × 35 cm (14 × 14″) portrait (see *Note*)
- Grid

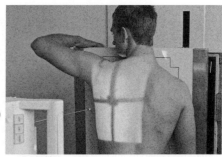

Fig. 7.13 45° RAO above diaphragm—bilateral, right anterior injury (to shift spine away from injury).

Position
- Erect (preferred), or recumbent if needed
- Oblique 45°, rotate spine away from area of interest
- Involved region of thorax is centered to IR.

Note: Some routines indicate unilateral oblique only of affected side with smaller IR placed portrait.

Central Ray: CR ⊥ to center of IR to level 7–8″ (18 to 20 cm) below vertebra prominens (T7)

SID: 72″ (183 cm) erect, 40″ (102 cm) recumbent

Collimation: Collimate to region of interest

Respiration: Above diaphragm—expose on **inspiration**

kV Range:		Analog: 70–80 kV			Digital Systems: 85 ± 5 kV		
	cm	kV	mA	Time	mAs	SID	Exposure Indicator
S							
M							
L							

Bontrager Textbook, 9th ed, p. 371.

Bony Thorax

7

Posterior Oblique (LPO): Lower Axillary Ribs

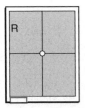

- 35 × 43 cm (14 × 17″) or 35 × 35 cm (14 × 14″) portrait
- Grid

Position
- Erect or recumbent (recumbent preferred)
- Top of IR ≈1.5″ (4 cm) above shoulders
- Rotate 45° from AP, arm closest to IR up, resting on head; opposite hand on waist with arm away from body

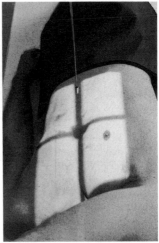

Fig. 7.14 45° LPO (below diaphragm).

Central Ray: CR ⊥ centered to IR to level midway between xiphoid process and lower rib margin

SID: 72″ (183 cm) erect, 40″ (102 cm) recumbent

Collimation: Collimate to region of interest

Respiration: Below diaphragm—expose upon **expiration**

Bony Thorax

7

kV Range:		Analog: 70–80 kV			Digital Systems: 85 ± 5 kV		
	cm	kV	mA	Time	mAs	SID	Exposure Indicator
S							
M							
L							

Anterior or Posterior Oblique: Axillary Ribs
Above and Below Diaphragm

Evaluation Criteria

Anatomy Demonstrated

- **LPO/RAO:** Visualizes (elongates) left axillary ribs
- **RPO/LAO:** Visualizes (elongates) right axillary ribs
- Ribs 1–9 seen above diaphragm
- Ribs 10–12 seen below diaphragm (minimum)
- Axillary portion of ribs projected without superimposition

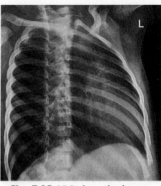

Fig. 7.15 LPO above diaphragm.

Competency Check: _____
Technologist   Date

Position

- 45° oblique should visualize axillary ribs in profile with spine shifted away from area of interest

Exposure

- No motion, sharp bony margins
- Optimal contrast and density (brightness) visualizes ribs through lungs and heart shadow for above diaphragm, and through dense abdominal organs for below diaphragm

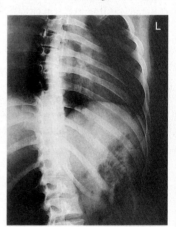

Fig. 7.16 LPO below diaphragm.

Competency Check: _____
Technologist   Date

Chapter 8

Cranium, Facial Bones, and Paranasal Sinuses

Cranium, Facial Bones, and Paranasal Sinuses

8

225

(R) Routine, (S) Special

8

Cranial Positioning Lines and Landmarks

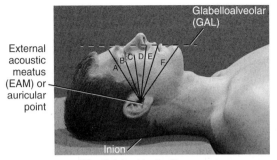

Fig. 8.1 Positioning lines.

A. Glabellomeatal line (**GML**)
B. Orbitomeatal line (**OML**)
C. Infraorbitomeatal line (**IOML**) (Reid's base line, or "base line," base of cranium)
D. Acanthiomeatal line (**AML**)
E. Lips-meatal line (**LML**) (used for modified Waters)
F. Mentomeatal line (**MML**) (used for Waters)

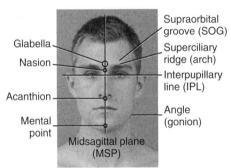

Fig. 8.2 Cranial landmarks.

- **Common positioning errors:** Rotation, tilt, flexion, and extension errors are the most common seen with cranial and facial bone radiography. See p. 409 in text to review these positioning errors and corrections.
- **Shielding:** All radiosensitive tissues outside the region of interest should be shielded during each imaging series.

Remove all metal, plastic, or other removable objects from the patient's head.

AP Axial: Cranium
Towne Method

- 24 × 30 cm (10 × 12″) portrait
- Grid

Position
- Seated erect, or supine, midsagittal plane aligned to CR and midline of the table and/or IR, perpendicular to IR; no rotation or tilt
- Depress chin to bring OML or IOML perpendicular to IR
- Center IR to projecting CR

Central Ray:
- CR 30° caudad to OML; or 37° caudad to IOML
- CR to ≈2.5″ (6.5 cm) above glabella (through 0.75″ [2 cm] superior to level of EAMs)

SID: 40″ (102 cm)

Collimation: On four sides to skull margins

Respiration: Suspend during exposure

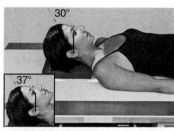

Fig. 8.3 AP axial (Towne)—CR 30° caudad to OML.

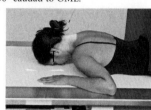

Fig. 8.4 PA axial (Haas method), OML ⊥ CR 25° cephalad, through level of EAMs.

Note: PA Axial—Haas method (p. 418 in text) is an alternative to AP Towne. Adjust head to bring OML ⊥ to IR. CR is angled 25° cephalad and exits 1½″ (4 cm) superior to nasion.

---

8 | kV Range: | Analog: 75–85 kV | Digital Systems: 80–90 kV |

	cm	kV	mA	Time	mAs	SID	Exposure Indicator
S							
M							
L							

Bontrager Textbook, 9th ed, p. 413.

AP Axial (Towne Method): Cranium

Evaluation Criteria

Anatomy Demonstrated

- Occipital bone, petrous pyramids, and foramen magnum

Position

- Dorsum sellae within foramen magnum
- **No rotation** evident by symmetry of petrous portion (pyramids) of temporal bones

Exposure

- Optimal density (brightness) and contrast to visualize occipital bone and structures within foramen magnum
- Sharp bony margins; no motion

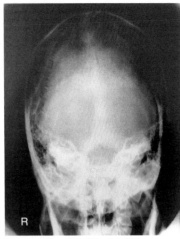

Fig. 8.5 AP axial skull.

Competency Check: _____

Technologist　　　　　Date

8

Lateral: Cranium

- 24 × 30 cm (10 × 12″) landscape
- Grid

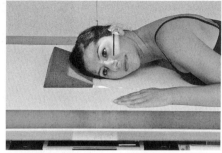

Fig. 8.6 Lateral skull.

Position
- Seated erect or semiprone on table
- Head in true lateral position, no rotation or tilt, midsagittal plane parallel to IR, and IPL perpendicular to IR
- Adjust chin to place IOML parallel to upper and lower IR edges
- Center IR to CR

Central Ray: CR ⊥ to IR, ≈2″ (5 cm) superior to EAM

SID: 40″ (102 cm)

Collimation: On four sides to skull margins

Respiration: Suspend during exposure

kV Range:	Analog: 70–80 kV			Digital Systems: 75–85 kV		
	cm	kV	mA	Time	mAs	SID	Exposure Indicator
S							
M							
L							

Bontrager Textbook, 9th ed, p. 414.

8

Lateral: Cranium

Evaluation Criteria

Anatomy Demonstrated

- Entire cranium visualized and superimposed cranial halves
- Entire sella turcica and dorsum sellae

Position

- **No tilt,** evident by superimposition of orbital plates (roofs)
- **No rotation,** evident by superimposition of greater wings of sphenoid and mandibular rami

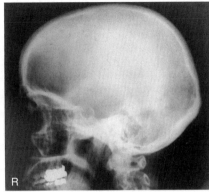

Fig. 8.7 Lateral skull.

Competency Check: _____
Technologist   Date

Exposure

- Optimal density (brightness) and contrast to visualize sellar structures
- Sharp bony margins; no motion

8

PA and PA Axial (15°): Cranium
Caldwell Method

Note: Some departmental routines include a PA to better demonstrate the frontal bone in addition to the 15° PA axial (Caldwell).

- 24 × 30 cm (10 × 12″) portrait
- Grid

Position

- Seated erect, or prone on table, head aligned to CR and midline of the table and/or IR
- With patient's forehead and nose resting on tabletop, adjust head to place OML perpendicular to IR
- No rotation or tilt, midsagittal plane perpendicular to IR
- Center IR to projected CR

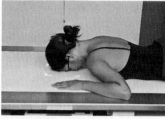

Fig. 8.8 PA—0°.

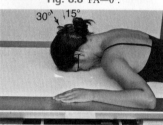

Fig. 8.9 PA axial—15° Caldwell.

Central Ray:

- **PA:** CR ⊥ to IR, centered to exit at glabella
- **PA axial (Caldwell):** CR 15° caudad to OML, centered to exit at nasion (25°–30° caudad best demonstrates orbital margins)

SID: 40″ (102 cm)

Collimation: On four sides to skull margins

Respiration: Suspend during exposure

kV Range:		Analog: 75–85 kV			Digital Systems: 80–90 kV	

	cm	kV	mA	Time	mAs	SID	Exposure Indicator
S							
M							
L							

Bontrager Textbook, 9th ed, p. 415.

Cranium, Facial Bones, and Paranasal Sinuses

8

PA and PA Axial (15°): Cranium
Caldwell Method

Evaluation Criteria
Anatomy Demonstrated
- **PA:** Frontal bone and crista galli demonstrated without distortion
- **PA axial 15°:** Greater/lesser wings of sphenoid, frontal bone, and superior orbital fissures

Position
- **PA:** Petrous ridges at level of superior orbital margin. No rotation; equal distance between orbits and lateral skull
- **PA axial 15°:** Petrous ridges projected in lower $\frac{1}{3}$ of orbits. No rotation; equal distance between orbits and lateral skull

Exposure
- Optimal density (brightness) and contrast to visualize frontal bone and surrounding structures
- Sharp bony margins; no motion

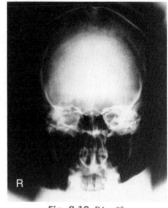

Fig. 8.10 PA—0°.

Competency Check: _____
                           Technologist   Date

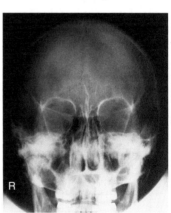

Fig. 8.11 PA axial—15° Caldwell.

Competency Check: _____
                           Technologist   Date

Submentovertical (SMV): Cranium

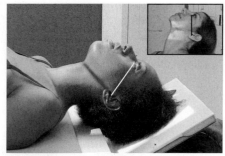

Fig. 8.12 SMV—CR ⊥ to IOML.

- 24 × 30 cm (10 × 12″) portrait
- Grid
- AEC optional

Position

- Seated erect or supine with head extended over end of table resting top of head against grid IR (may tilt table up slightly). A positioning sponge/pillow may be placed under shoulders
- Adjust IR and hyperextend neck to place IOML parallel to IR
- Ensure no rotation or tilt
- Center IR to CR

Central Ray: CR angled to be ⊥ to IOML, centered to 0.75″ (2 cm) anterior to level of EAMs (midpoint between angles of mandible)

Note: If patient cannot extend head this far, adjust CR as needed to remain perpendicular to IOML.

SID: 40″ (102 cm)

Collimation: On four sides to skull margins

Respiration: Suspend during exposure

---

8 kV Range: Analog: 75–85 kV Digital Systems: 80–90 kV

	cm	kV	mA	Time	mAs	SID	Exposure Indicator
S							
M							
L							

Bontrager Textbook, 9th ed, p. 417.

SMV: Cranium

Evaluation Criteria
Anatomy Demonstrated
- Foramen ovale and spinosum, mandible, sphenoid and posterior ethmoid sinuses, mastoid processes, petrous ridges, hard palate, foramen magnum, and occipital bone

Position
- Mandibular condyles are anterior to the petrous portion of temporal bone
- **No tilt;** equal distance between mandibular condyles and lateral skull
- **No rotation;** MSP parallel to edge of radiograph

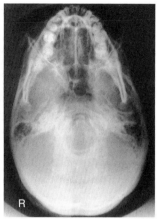

Fig. 8.13 SMV.

Competency Check: _____
Technologist   Date

Exposure
- Optimal density (brightness) and contrast to visualize outline of foramen magnum
- Sharp bony margins; no motion

8

Lateral: Cranium (Trauma)

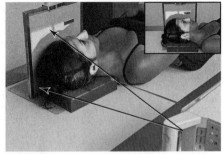

Fig. 8.14 Lateral, with possible spinal injury.

Warning: Do **NOT** elevate or move patient's head before cervical spine injuries have been ruled out.

- 24 × 30 cm (10 × 12") landscape (aligned to the anterior-to-posterior dimension of the skull)
- Grid

Position

- Supine, without removing cervical collar, if present
- With possible spinal injury, move patient to back edge of table and place IR about 1" (2.5 cm) below tabletop and posterior skull (move floating tabletop forward)
- Place head in true lateral position
- Center IR to horizontal beam CR (to include entire skull)
- Ensure no rotation or tilt

Central Ray: CR horizontal, ⊥ to IR, centered to ≈2" (5 cm) superior to EAM

SID: 40" (102 cm)

Collimation: On four sides to skull margins

Respiration: Suspend respiration

---

8 kV Range: Analog: 70–80 kV   Digital Systems: 75–85 kV

	cm	kV	mA	Time	mAs	SID	Exposure Indicator
S							
M							
L							

AP and AP Axial: Skull (Trauma)

Warning: With possible spine or severe head injuries, perform all projections AP without moving patient's head or without removing cervical collar unless requested to do so by physician.

- 24 × 30 cm (10 × 12″) portrait
- Grid (bucky)

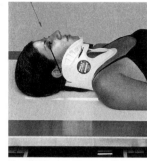

Fig. 8.15 AP, CR—parallel to OML—centered to glabella.

Position

- Patient carefully moved onto x-ray table in supine position
- All projections performed as is, without moving patient's head

SID: 40″ (102 cm)

Collimation: On four sides to skull margins

Respiration: Suspend during exposure

CR Angle and Centering

- As indicated in Figs. 8.15, 8.16 and 8.17
- IR centered to projected CR

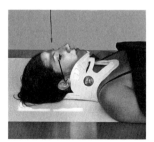

Fig. 8.16 AP reverse Caldwell. CR—15° cephalad to OML—centered to nasion.

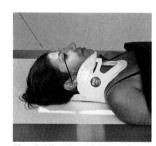

Fig. 8.17 AP axial (Towne). CR—30° caudad to OML—CR to ≈2.5″ (5–6 cm) above glabella.

Lateral: Skull (Trauma)

Evaluation Criteria

Anatomy Demonstrated

- Entire cranium and superimposed cranial halves
- Entire sella turcica and dorsum sellae

Position

- No rotation or tilt (see p. 237 for specific criteria)

Exposure

- Optimal density (brightness) and contrast to visualize sellar structures
- Sharp bony margins; no motion

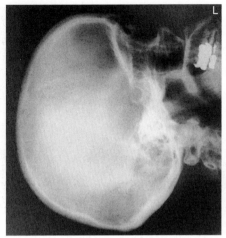

Fig. 8.18 Lateral trauma skull.

Competency Check: _____

Technologist   Date

AP and AP Axial: Skull (Trauma)

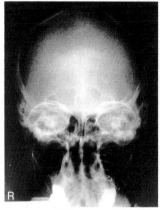

Fig. 8.19 AP to OML.

Competency Check: _____
           Technologist   Date

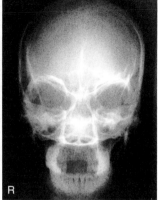

Fig. 8.20 AP axial ("reverse") Caldwell) (15° cephalad).

Competency Check: _____
           Technologist   Date

Evaluation Criteria

Anatomy Demonstrated

- **AP 0°:** Frontal bone and crista galli demonstrated (magnified because of OID)
- **AP axial 15°:** Greater/lesser wings of sphenoid, frontal bone, and superior orbital fissures

Position

- **AP 0°:** Petrous ridges at level of superior orbital margin.
  No rotation; equal distance between orbits and lateral skull
- **AP axial 15°:** Petrous ridges projected in lower ⅓ of orbits.
  No rotation; equal distance between orbits and lateral skull

Exposure

- Optimal density (brightness) and contrast to visualize frontal bone and surrounding structures
- Sharp bony margins; no motion

Lateral: Facial Bones

- 18 × 24 cm (8 × 10″) portrait
- Grid

Position
- Erect or semiprone on table
- Adjust head to true lateral position with side of interest closest to IR

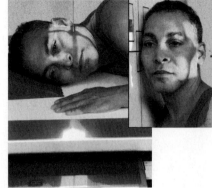

Fig. 8.21 Lateral facial bones.

- No rotation or tilt, midsagittal plane parallel to IR, IPL perpendicular to IR
- Adjust chin to place IOML parallel to top and bottom edge of IR
- Center IR to CR

Central Ray: CR ⊥ to IR, to zygoma (prominence of the cheek) midway between EAM and outer canthus
SID: 40″ (102 cm)
Collimation: On four sides to area of facial bones
Respiration: Suspend during exposure

---

8 kV Range: Analog: 65–75 kV   Digital Systems: 70–80 kV

	cm	kV	mA	Time	mAs	SID	Exposure Indicator
S							
M							
L							

Lateral: Facial Bones

Evaluation Criteria

Anatomy Demonstrated
- Superimposed facial bones, greater wings of sphenoid and sella turcica
- Region from orbital roofs to mentum demonstrated

Position
- **No tilt;** evident by superimposition of orbital plates (roofs)
- **No rotation;** evident by superimposition of greater wings of sphenoid and mandibular rami

Exposure
- Optimal density (brightness) and contrast to visualize facial structures
- Sharp bony margins; no motion

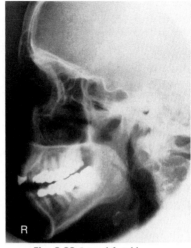

Fig. 8.22 Lateral facial bones.

Competency Check: _____
                  Technologist   Date

Parietoacanthial: Facial Bones
Waters and Modified Waters Methods

- 18 × 24 cm (8 × 10″) portrait or 24 × 30 cm (10 × 12″) portrait
- Grid

Position
Waters
- Seated erect or prone on table (erect preferred)
- Extend head resting on chin; place MML ⊥ to IR, which places the OML 37° to IR
- Center IR to CR

Modified Waters
- OML is 55° to the plane of the IR, or line from junction of lips to EAM (LML) is ⊥ to IR

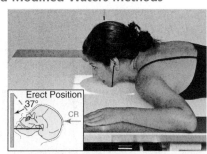

Fig. 8.23 PA Waters, OML 37°—CR and MML ⊥.

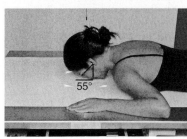

Fig. 8.24 PA modified Waters, OML 55°—CR and LML ⊥.

Central Ray: CR ⊥ to IR, to exit at acanthion (both projections)
SID: 40″ (102 cm)
Collimation: On four sides to area of facial bones
Respiration: Suspend during exposure

	cm	kV	mA	Time	mAs	SID	Exposure Indicator
kV Range:		Analog: 70–80 kV			Digital Systems: 75–85 kV		
S							
M							
L							

Bontrager Textbook, 9th ed, pp. 420 and 422.

Parietoacanthial and Modified Parietoacanthial
Waters and Modified Waters Methods

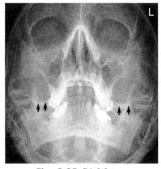

Fig. 8.25 PA Waters.

Competency Check: _____
Technologist   Date

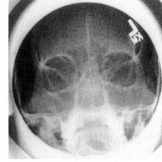

Fig. 8.26 PA modified Waters.

Competency Check: _____
Technologist   Date

Cranium, Facial Bones, and Paranasal Sinuses

Evaluation Criteria

Anatomy Demonstrated
- **Waters:** General survey of facial bones; inferior orbital rims, maxillae, and nasal septum
- **Modified Waters:** Inferior orbital floors in profile (undistorted). Ideal projection to demonstrate possible "blow out" fractures of orbital floor

Position
- **Waters:** Petrous ridges just inferior to floor of maxillary sinuses. **No rotation;** equal distance between orbits and lateral skull
- **Modified Waters:** Petrous ridges projected in lower $\frac{1}{2}$ of maxillary sinuses. **No rotation;** equal distance between orbits and lateral skull

Exposure
- Optimal density (brightness) and contrast to visualize maxillary region and surrounding structures
- Sharp bony margins; no motion

8

243

PA Axial (15°): Facial Bones
Caldwell Method

- 18 × 24 cm (8 × 10″) portrait or 24 × 30 cm (10 × 12″) portrait
- Grid

Position
- Seated erect or prone on table, MSP aligned to CR and to midline of the table and/or IR
- With forehead and nose resting on

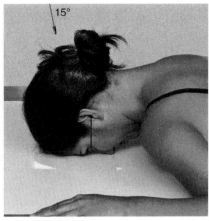

Fig. 8.27 PA axial—15° Caldwell (OML ⊥); CR to exit at nasion.

imaging device, adjust head to place OML perpendicular to IR; ensure no rotation or tilt
- Center IR to projected CR (to nasion)

Central Ray: CR 15° caudal to OML, centered to exit at nasion

Note: A 30° CR angle is required to project petrous ridges below lower orbital margins if this is an area of interest. CR will exit at level of midorbits

SID: 40″ (102 cm)

Collimation: On four sides to skull (facial bones) margins

Respiration: Suspend during exposure

---

kV Range:		Analog: 70–80 kV			Digital Systems: 75–85 kV		
	cm	kV	mA	Time	mAs	SID	Exposure Indicator
S							
M							
L							

Bontrager Textbook, 9th ed, p. 421.

PA Axial (15°): Facial Bones
Caldwell Method

Evaluation Criteria
Anatomy Demonstrated
- Orbital rims, maxillae, nasal septum, and zygomatic arches

Position
- Petrous ridges projected in lower $\frac{1}{3}$ of orbits. **No rotation;** equal distance between orbits and lateral skull margins

Exposure
- Optimal density (brightness) and contrast to visualize maxillary region and orbital floor
- Sharp bony margins; no motion

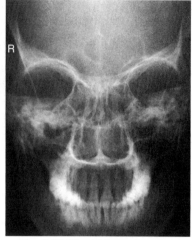

Fig. 8.28 PA axial Caldwell—15° caudad.

Competency Check: _____
　　　　　　　　　　　Technologist　　　　　Date

Lateral, Acanthioparietal: Facial Bones (Trauma)
Reverse Waters and Reverse Modified Waters Methods

Warning: With possible spine or severe head injuries, perform all projections with patient supine without moving patient's head or without removing cervical collar, if present.

Lateral (Horizontal Beam)
- 18 × 24 cm (8 × 10″) portrait
- Grid, placed on edge against lateral cranium
- Ensure no rotation or tilt, MSP parallel to IR
- CR horizontal, to midway between outer canthus and EAM

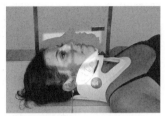

Fig. 8.29 Horizontal beam lateral—CR to midway between outer canthus and EAM.

Reverse Waters
- 18 × 24 cm (8 × 10″) portrait
- Grid (bucky), AEC—center field
- MSP aligned to CR and midline of table or IR
- Ensure no rotation or tilt
- CR parallel to MML
- CR centered to acanthion (CR angled cephalad, as needed, unless cervical injury has been ruled out)

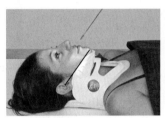

Fig. 8.30 Trauma reverse Waters—CR parallel to MML, centered to acanthion.

Reverse Modified Waters
- Same as reverse Waters except:
  - CR parallel to junction of lips-meatal line (LML)
  - CR centered to acanthion

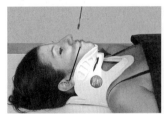

Fig. 8.31 Trauma reverse modified Waters—CR parallel to LML, centered to acanthion.

Parieto-Orbital Oblique: Optic Foramina
Rhese Method

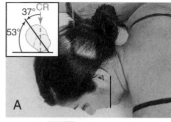

- 18 × 24 cm (8 × 10″) landscape
- Grid
- Bilateral orbit study performed for comparison
- AEC not recommended

Position

- Seated erect or prone on table
- As a starting reference, adjust the head so the nose, cheek, and chin are touching the tabletop
- Adjust the head so the plane of AML is perpendicular to the IR, and the midsagittal plane is 53° to the IR (use angle indicator)
- Center IR to CR (to downside orbit)

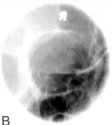

Fig. 8.32 A, Rhese oblique (right side). **B**, Rhese oblique.
—AML and CR ⊥
—53° rotation of head from lateral

Central Ray: CR ⊥ to IR, to midportion of downside orbit
SID: 40″ (102 cm)
Collimation: Closely collimate to 3–4″ (8–10 cm) square
Respiration: Suspend during exposure

kV Range: Analog: 70–80 kV   Digital Systems: 75–85 kV

	cm	kV	mA	Time	mAs	SID	Exposure Indicator
S							
M							
L							

Cranium, Facial Bones, and Paranasal Sinuses

8

Bilateral SMV: Zygomatic Arches

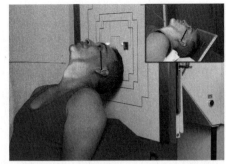

- 24 × 30 cm (10 × 12″) landscape
- Grid
- AEC not recommended

Position

- Seated erect or supine with head extended over end

Fig. 8.33 SMV, bilateral zygomatic arches, erect—CR ⊥ to IOML (nongrid may be preferred).

of table resting top of head against grid IR (table may be tilted up slightly)
- Adjust IR and head to place IOML parallel to IR
- Ensure no rotation or tilt
- Center IR to CR

Central Ray: CR angled as needed to be ⊥ to IOML, centered to midway between zygomatic arches (≈1.5″ or 4 cm inferior to mandibular symphysis)

SID: 40″ (102 cm)

Collimation: To include area of zygomatic arches

Respiration: Suspend during exposure

	cm	kV	mA	Time	mAs	SID	Exposure Indicator
S							
M							
L							

kV Range: Analog: 70–80 kV   Digital Systems: 75–85 kV

8

Oblique Inferosuperior (Tangential): Zygomatic Arches

Bilateral arches generally taken for comparison.

- 18 × 24 cm (8 × 10″) portrait
- Grid
- AEC not recommended

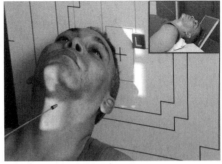

Fig. 8.34 Tangential of left zygomatic arch—CR ⊥ to IOML, head tilted 15°, rotated 15°.

Position

- Position as for an SMV skull with the IOML parallel to the IR
- **Rotate** the head ≈15° **toward** side being examined
- **Tilt** the midsagittal plane ≈15° **toward** the side being examined (more tilt may be needed to free the zygomatic arch from superimposition by mandible or parietal bone)
- Center IR to CR

Central Ray: CR angled if needed to be ⊥ to IOML, centered to midzygomatic arch

SID: 40″ (102 cm)

Collimation: Collimate closely to area of interest

Respiration: Suspend during exposure

---

kV Range: Analog: 70–80 kV   Digital Systems: 75–85 kV   ∞

	cm	kV	mA	Time	mAs	SID	Exposure Indicator
S							
M							
L							

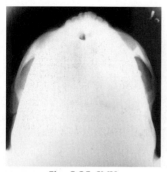

Fig. 8.35 SMV.

Competency Check: _____

             Technologist   Date

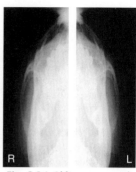

Fig. 8.36 Oblique tangential.

Competency Check: _____

             Technologist Date

Evaluation Criteria

Anatomy Demonstrated

- **SMV:** Bilateral zygomatic arches
- **Tangential:** Unilateral zygomatic arch

Position

- **SMV:** Unobstructed view of bilateral arches. No rotation; symmetry of arches
- **Oblique inferosuperior (tangential):** Unilateral view of unobstructed arch. No superimposition of arch with parietal bone or mandible

Exposure

- Optimal density (brightness) and contrast to visualize the zygomatic arches
- Sharp bony margins with soft tissue detail; no motion

8

AP Axial: Zygomatic Arches
Modified Towne Method

- 18 × 24 cm (8 × 10″) landscape
- Grid
- AEC not recommended

Position
- Seated erect or supine on table, midsagittal plane aligned to midline of table or IR; ensure no rotation or tilt
- Depress chin to bring either the OML or the IOML perpendicular to IR
- Center IR to projected CR

Central Ray:
- CR 30° caudad to OML; or 37° to IOML
- CR 1″ (2.5 cm) superior to nasion to pass through level of midarches

SID: 40″ (102 cm)
Collimation: On four sides to area of bilateral arches
Respiration: Suspend during exposure

Fig. 8.37 **A,** AP axial—CR 37° to IOML. **B,** AP axial.

Cranium, Facial Bones, and Paranasal Sinuses

kV Range:	Analog: 70–80 kV	Digital Systems: 75–85 kV	8

	cm	kV	mA	Time	mAs	SID	Exposure Indicator
S							
M							
L							

Lateral: Nasal Bones

Bilateral projections generally taken for comparison.

- 18×24 cm ($8 \times 10''$) landscape
- Nongrid—detail screens (analog)

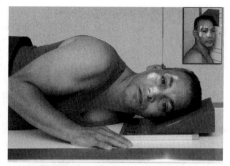

Fig. 8.38 Left lateral—nasal bones.

Position

- Seated erect or semiprone on table
- Center nasal bones to half of IR and to CR
- Adjust head to bring IOML parallel to top and bottom edge of IR
- Ensure a true lateral, IPL perpendicular to IR, and midsagittal plane parallel to IR

Central Ray: CR ⊥ to IR, centered to ≈0.5″ (1.25 cm) inferior to nasion

SID: 40″ (102 cm)

Collimation: Closely collimate to ≈4″ (10 cm) square

Respiration: Suspend during exposure

8

kV Range:	Analog: 60–70 kV			Digital Systems: 65–75 kV		
	cm	kV	mA	Time	mAs	SID	Exposure Indicator
S							
M							
L							

Lateral: Nasal Bones

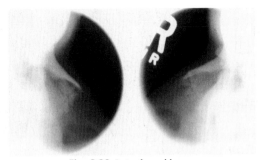

Fig. 8.39 Lateral nasal bones.

Competency Check: _____

Technologist   Date

Evaluation Criteria

Anatomy Demonstrated

- Nasal bones with soft tissue structures
- Frontonasal suture to anterior nasal spine

Position

- **No rotation;** complete profile of nasal bones
- Frontonasal suture to anterior nasal spine within collimation field

Exposure

- Optimal density (brightness) and contrast to visualize nasal bones and surrounding soft tissue structures
- Sharp bony margins with soft tissue detail; no motion

Superoinferior Tangential (Axial): Nasal Bones

Cranium, Facial Bones, and Paranasal Sinuses

- 18 × 24 cm (8 × 10″) landscape
- Nongrid—detail screens (analog)

Position
- Seated erect at end of table or prone on table
- If prone, place supports under chest and under IR
- Rest extended chin on IR, which should be perpendicular to GAL (glabelloalveolar line) and to CR

Central Ray: CR directed parallel to GAL, tangential to the glabella

SID: 40″ (102 cm)

Collimation: Closely collimate to ≈4″ (10 cm) square

Respiration: Suspend during exposure

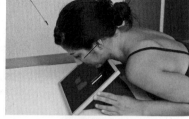

Fig. 8.40 Seated.

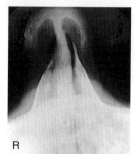

R

Fig. 8.41 Superoinferior.

kV Range:		Analog: 60–70 kV			Digital Systems: 70–80 kV		
	cm	kV	mA	Time	mAs	SID	Exposure Indicator
S							
M							
L							

Bontrager Textbook, 9th ed, p. 424.

PA and PA Axial: Mandible

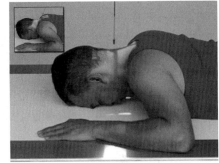

- 18 × 24 cm (8 × 10")
  or 24 × 30 cm
  (10 × 12") portrait
- Grid
- AEC not
  recommended

Fig. 8.42 PA mandible—CR and OML ⊥ to IR.)

Position
- Seated erect or
  prone on table,
  head aligned to midline of the table and/or IR
- With forehead and nose resting on tabletop, adjust head to place OML ⊥ to IR
- No rotation or tilt, midsagittal plane ⊥ to IR
- Center IR to CR (level of junction of lips)

Central Ray: CR ⊥ to IR, to exit at level of lips

PA Axial (Optional): A CR angle of 20°–25° cephalad centered to exit at the acanthion best demonstrates proximal rami and condyles

SID: 40" (102 cm)

Collimation: Collimate to area of mandible (square area)

Respiration: Suspend during exposure

Cranium, Facial Bones, and Paranasal Sinuses

	cm	kV	mA	Time	mAs	SID	Exposure Indicator
S							
M							
L							

kV Range: Analog: 75–85 kV   Digital Systems: 80–90 kV   8

Axiolateral and Axiolateral Oblique: Mandible

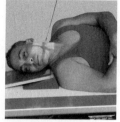

Fig. 8.43 Semisupine.

Fig. 8.44 Erect axiolateral oblique.

R and L sides generally imaged for comparison unless contraindicated.

- 18 × 24 cm (8 × 10″) or 24 × 30 cm (10 × 12″) landscape
- Grid or nongrid
- AEC not recommended

—CR 25° cephalad (maximum)
—10°–15° head rotation for general survey (as shown above)
—0° head rotation for ramus
—30° head rotation for body
—45° head rotation for mentum

Position

- Seated erect, semiprone, or semisupine, with support under shoulder and hip
- Extend chin, with side of interest against IR
- Adjust head so IPL is perpendicular to IR, no tilt
- Rotate head toward IR as determined by area of interest
  - Head in true lateral demonstrates ramus (axiolateral)
  - 10°–15° rotation best provides a general survey of the mandible
  - 30° rotation toward IR best demonstrates body
  - 45° rotation best demonstrates mentum

Central Ray: CR 25° cephalad to IPL, centered to downside midmandible (≈2″ or 5 cm below upside angle)
SID: 40″ (102 cm)
Collimation: To area of mandible (square area)
Respiration: Suspend during exposure

kV Range:	Analog: 70–80 kV				Digital Systems: 75–85 kV	
	cm	kV	mA	Time	mAs	SID	Exposure Indicator
S							
M							
L							

Bontrager Textbook, 9th ed, p. 429.

Axiolateral Oblique: Mandible (Trauma)

For trauma patients unable to cooperate.
- 18 × 24 cm (8 × 10″) or 24 × 30 cm (10 × 12″) landscape
- Grid or nongrid

Position
- Supine, no rotation of head, MSP ⊥ to tabletop
- IR on edge next to face, parallel to MSP with lower edge of IR ≈1″ (2.5 cm) below lower border of mandible
- Depress shoulders and elevate or extend chin, if possible

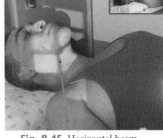

Fig. 8.45 Horizontal beam axiolateral—CR 25° cephalad from lateral, 5°–10° down.

Note: May rotate head toward IR slightly (10°–15°) to better visualize body or mentum of mandible if this is area of interest.

Central Ray:
- CR horizontal beam, 25° cephalad (from lateral or IPL); angled down (posteriorly) 5°–10° to clear shoulder
- CR centered to ≈2″ (5 cm) distal to angle of mandible on side away from IR

SID: 40″ (102 cm)

Collimation: To area of mandible (square area)

Respiration: Suspend during exposure

| kV Range: | Analog: 70–80 kV | | Digital Systems: 75–85 kV |

	cm	kV	mA	Time	mAs	SID	Exposure Indicator
S							
M							
L							

Cranium, Facial Bones, and Paranasal Sinuses

8

PA and Axiolateral Oblique: Mandible

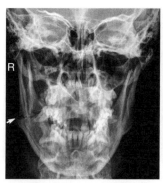

Fig. 8.46 PA mandible.
Competency Check: _____
Technologist   Date

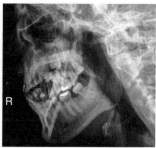

Fig. 8.47 Axiolateral oblique mandible.
Competency Check: _____
Technologist   Date

Evaluation Criteria

Anatomy Demonstrated
- **PA:** Mandibular rami and lateral portion of body
- **Axiolateral and Axiolateral Oblique:** Mandibular rami, condylar and coronoid processes, and body of near side

Position
- **PA: No rotation** evident by symmetry of rami
- **Axiolateral and Axiolateral Oblique:** Unobstructed view of mandibular rami, body, and mentum. No foreshortening of area of interest

Exposure
- Optimal density (brightness) and contrast to visualize mandibular area of interest
- Sharp bony margins; no motion

AP Axial: Mandible or Temporomandibular Joints and Condyloid Processes

- 18 × 24 cm (8 × 10″) or 24 × 30 cm (10 × 12″) portrait
- Grid

Position

- Seated erect or supine on table, midsagittal plane centered to midline of table; ensure no rotation or tilt

Fig. 8.48 AP axial, CR 35° to OML (CR centered for mandible).

- Depress chin to bring OML perpendicular to IR, if possible (or place IOML perpendicular and add 7° to CR angle)
- Center IR to projected CR

Central Ray:
- CR 35° to OML (42° to IOML) caudad
- CR centered to glabella for mandible

Note: CR centered ≈1″ (2.5 cm) above glabella to pass through TMJs if TMJs are of primary interest

SID: 40″ (102 cm)

Collimation: To include from TMJs to body of mandible

Respiration: Suspend during exposure

Cranium, Facial Bones, and Paranasal Sinuses

kV Range:	Analog: 75–85 kV		Digital Systems: 80–90 kV			8

	cm	kV	mA	Time	mAs	SID	Exposure Indicator
S							
M							
L							

Axiolateral Oblique: Temporomandibular Joints
Modified Law Method

Bilateral sides imaged for comparison in both open and closed mouth positions.
- 18 × 24 cm (8 × 10″) portrait (divided on same IR)
- Grid

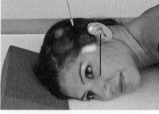

Fig. 8.49 Closed mouth.

Position
- Seated erect (preferred) or semiprone on table, affected side down
- Adjust chin to place IOML perpendicular to front edge of IR

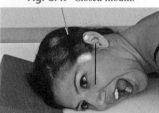

Fig. 8.50 Open mouth. —15° oblique (from lateral) and 15° CR (caudad)

- Rotate skull (midsagittal plane) 15° toward IR, no tilt, IPL remains perpendicular to IR
- Portion of IR being exposed centered to CR
- Second exposure in same position except with mouth fully open

Central Ray: CR 15° caudad, centered to enter 1½″ (4 cm) superior to upside EAM

SID: 40″ (102 cm)

Collimation: Collimate to 3–4″ (8–10 cm) square

Respiration: Suspend during exposure

	cm	kV	mA	Time	mAs	SID	Exposure Indicator
kV Range:		Analog: 75–85 kV			Digital Systems: 80–90 kV		
S							
M							
L							

Bontrager Textbook, 9th ed, p. 435.

Axiolateral: Temporomandibular Joints
Schuller Method

Bilateral sides imaged for comparison in both open and closed mouth positions.

- 18 × 24 cm (8 × 10″) portrait (divided on same IR)
- Grid

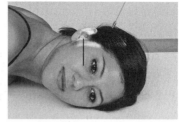

Fig. 8.51 Closed mouth.

Position

- Seated erect or semiprone, affected side down
- Adjust chin to place IOML perpendicular to front edge of IR, true lateral, no rotation or tilt of head
- Portion of IR being exposed centered to projected CR

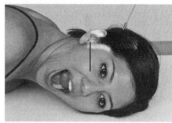

Fig. 8.52 Open mouth.
—25° caudad, 0° rotation

- Second exposure in same position except with mouth fully open

Central Ray: CR 25°–30° caudad, centered to enter 2″ (5 cm) superior and ½″ (1–2 cm) anterior to upside EAM

SID: 40″ (102 cm)

Collimation: Collimate to 3–4″ (8–10 cm) square

Respiration: Suspend during exposure

Cranium, Facial Bones, and Paranasal Sinuses

	cm	kV	mA	Time	mAs	SID	Exposure Indicator
S							
M							
L							

kV Range: Analog: 75–85 kV   Digital Systems: 80–90 kV   8

Axiolateral Oblique (Modified Law Method) and Axiolateral (Schuller Method): Temporomandibular Joints

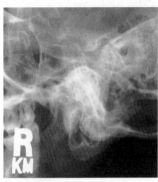

Fig. 8.53 Axiolateral oblique—closed mouth, downside TMJ shown in fossa (modified Law).

Competency Check: _____
                          Technologist   Date

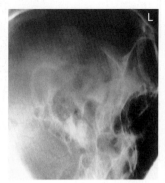

Fig. 8.54 Axiolateral projection—open mouth; TMJ shown with condyle moved to anterior margin of fossa (Schuller).

Competency Check: _____
                          Technologist   Date

Note: Positioning routine would require both open and closed mouth of modified Law method, or both open and closed of Schuller method.

Evaluation Criteria

Anatomy Demonstrated

- **Modified Law:** Bilateral, functional study of TMJ and fossa
- **Schuller:** Bilateral, functional study of TMJ and fossa

Position

- **Modified Law:** Unobstructed view of TMJ in both open and closed mouth positions (only closed mouth is shown)
- **Schuller:** Unobstructed view of TMJ in both open and closed mouth positions. Greater elongation of the condyles (only open mouth is shown)

Exposure

- Optimal density (brightness) and contrast to visualize the TMJ and mandibular fossa
- Sharp bony margins; no motion

Lateral: Paranasal Sinuses

Requires an **erect position with horizontal CR** to demonstrate air-fluid levels.

- 18 × 24 cm (8 × 10″) portrait
- Grid
- AEC not recommended

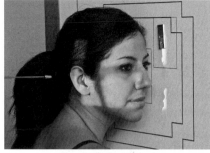

Fig. 8.55 Erect lateral.

Position

- Erect, seated facing IR, turn head into true lateral position
- Raise chin to bring IOML perpendicular to front edge of IR
- No rotation, midsagittal plane parallel and IPL ⊥ to IR
- Center IR to CR

Central Ray: CR horizontal to midway between EAM and outer canthus

SID: 40″ (102 cm)

Collimation: Collimate on four sides to region of sinuses

Respiration: Suspend during exposure

Cranium, Facial Bones, and Paranasal Sinuses

kV Range: Analog: 70–80 kV   Digital Systems: 75–85 kV   8

	cm	kV	mA	Time	mAs	SID	Exposure Indicator
S							
M							
L							

PA: Paranasal Sinuses
Modified PA–Caldwell Method

Requires an **erect position with horizontal CR** to demonstrate air-fluid levels.

- 18 × 24 cm (8 × 10″) portrait
- Grid
- AEC not recommended

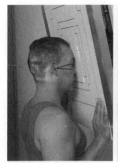

Fig. 8.56 PA Caldwell (if IR holder can be tilted).

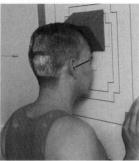

Fig. 8.57 Modified PA Caldwell (if IR holder cannot be tilted).

Position
PA Caldwell:
- Patient seated erect, facing IR; tilt top of IR 15° toward patient
- Adjust head so that OML is ⊥ to IR, no rotation
- IR centered to CR (nasion)

Modified PA Caldwell:
- Tilt head back to bring OML 15° from horizontal

Central Ray: CR horizontal (parallel to floor) and exits at nasion
SID: 40″ (102 cm)
Collimation: To region of sinuses
Respiration: Suspend during exposure

kV Range:		Analog: 75–85 kV		Digital Systems: 75–85 kV		

	cm	kV	mA	Time	mAs	SID	Exposure Indicator
S							
M							
L							

Bontrager Textbook, 9th ed, p. 438.

Lateral and PA (Modified Caldwell Method): Sinuses

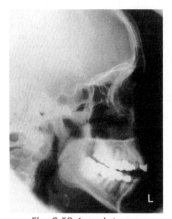

Fig. 8.58 Lateral sinuses.

Competency Check: _____
Technologist   Date

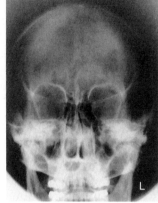

Fig. 8.59 PA axial (Caldwell method)—sinuses.

Competency Check: _____
Technologist   Date

Evaluation Criteria

Anatomy Demonstrated
- **Lateral:** All paranasal sinuses demonstrated
- **PA Caldwell:** Frontal and anterior ethmoid sinuses

Position
- **Lateral: No rotation or tilt;** superimposition of greater wings/ sphenoid, orbital roofs, and sella turcica
- **PA Caldwell:** Petrous ridges in lower $\frac{1}{3}$ of orbits. **No rotation;** equal distance between orbits and lateral skull

Exposure
- Optimal density (brightness) and contrast to visualize the paranasal sinuses
- Sharp bony margins with soft tissue detail; no motion

Parietoacanthial: Paranasal Sinuses
Waters Method

Requires an **erect position with horizontal CR** to demonstrate air-fluid levels.

- 18 × 24 cm (8 × 10")
  or 24 × 30 cm
  (10 × 12") portrait
- Grid
- AEC not recommended

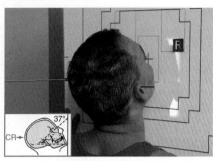

Fig. 8.60 PA erect Waters, MML ⊥, and CR horizontal.

Position
- Seated erect, chin extended and touching imaging device
- Adjust height of IR to center at acanthion
- Adjust MML perpendicular to IR (OML is 37° to IR)
- No rotation, midsagittal plane perpendicular to IR
- Center IR to CR

Optional Open-Mouth Position
- Patient opens mouth wide to better visualize sphenoid sinuses through the open mouth

Central Ray: CR horizontal and ⊥ to IR, to exit at acanthion
SID: 40" (102 cm)
Collimation: Collimate on four sides to area of sinuses
Respiration: Suspend during exposure

	kV Range:	Analog: 75–85 kV				Digital Systems: 75–85 kV	
	cm	kV	mA	Time	mAs	SID	Exposure Indicator
S							
M							
L							

8

Bontrager Textbook, 9th ed, p. 439.

SMV: Paranasal Sinuses

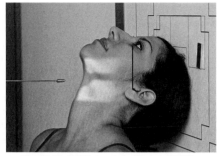

Requires an **erect position with horizontal CR** to demonstrate air-fluid levels.
- 18 × 24 cm (8 × 10″) or 24 × 30 cm (10 × 12″) portrait
- Grid
- AEC not recommended

Fig. 8.61 SMV sinuses—CR ⊥ to IOML and IR.

Position
- Seated erect, leaning back in chair and extending head to rest top of head against IR holder
- Adjust head to place IOML as near parallel to plane of IR as possible; ensure no rotation or tilt
- Center IR to CR

Central Ray: CR horizontal and ⊥ to IOML, centered to midpoint between angles of mandible at level 1½–2″ (4–5 cm) inferior to mandibular symphysis
SID: 40″ (102 cm)
Collimation: On four sides to region of sinuses
Respiration: Suspend during exposure

| kV Range: | Analog: 75–85 kV | | Digital Systems: 80–90 kV | | | 8 |

	cm	kV	mA	Time	mAs	SID	Exposure Indicator
S							
M							
L							

Parietoacanthial (Waters Method) and SMV: Sinuses

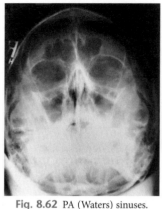

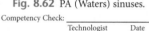

Fig. 8.62 PA (Waters) sinuses.

Competency Check: _____
                        Technologist   Date

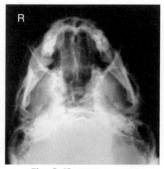

Fig. 8.63 SMV sinuses.

Competency Check: _____
                        Technologist   Date

Evaluation Criteria

Anatomy Demonstrated

- **Waters:** Unobstructed view of maxillary sinuses
- **SMV:** Unobstructed view of sphenoid, maxillary, and ethmoid sinuses

Position

- **Waters:** Petrous ridges just inferior to floor of maxillary sinuses. **No rotation;** equal distance between orbits and lateral skull
- **SMV:** Mandibular condyles projected anterior to petrous bone. **No rotation or tilt;** symmetry of petrous pyramids and equal distance between mandibular border and lateral skull

Exposure

- Optimal density (brightness) and contrast to visualize the paranasal sinuses
- Sharp bony margins with soft tissue detail; no motion

Chapter 9

Abdomen and Common Contrast Media Procedures

- Shielding and positioning landmarks......................... 271
- Barium distribution and body positions 272
- Acute Abdomen Series 273

Abdomen and Common Contrast Media Procedures

9

(R) Routine, (S) Special

Shielding and Positioning Landmarks

Shielding

All radiosensitive tissues outside the anatomy of interest should be shielded.

Gonadal Shielding

Males: Gonadal shields should be used on **all** males of reproductive age, with upper edge of shield placed at symphysis pubis unless it obscures essential anatomy.

Females: Ovarian gonadal shields may be used for abdomen examinations on all females, only **if** such shields do not obscure essential anatomy for that examination as determined by a radiologist/physician (shielding is especially important for children).

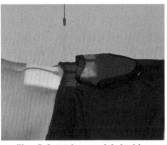

Fig. 9.1 Male gonadal shield (top of shield at symphysis pubis).

Pregnancy

Generally, no radiographic procedures exposing the pelvic region should be performed during pregnancy without special instruction from a radiologist/ physician.

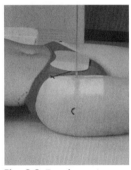

Fig. 9.2 Female ovarian shield (top of shield at or slightly above the level of ASIS, lower border just above symphysis pubis).

Topographic Positioning Landmarks

Certain positioning landmarks are essential for positioning the general abdomen and specific organs within the abdomen because the borders of these organs and the upper and lower margins of the general abdomen itself are not visible from the exterior.

Abdominal borders and organ locations, however, can be determined by certain landmarks, which can be located by gentle palpation with the fingertips, being careful of painful or sensitive areas. (The patient should be informed of the purpose for this before beginning the palpation process.)

Barium Distribution and Body Positions

The air-barium distribution within the stomach and large intestine changes with various body positions. By knowing these distribution patterns, one can determine the body position a radiograph was taken. Air always rises to the highest levels, and the heavy barium settles to the lowest levels (air is black, and barium is white).

Stomach

The fundus is located more posteriorly; therefore in the supine position, the fundus would be the lowest portion of the stomach and would be filled with barium.

In both prone and erect positions, the fundus would be filled with air, as seen on the drawings below, with a straight air-barium line on the erect.

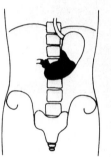 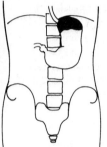 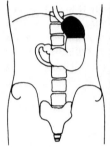

Fig. 9.3 Supine (barium in fundus).

Fig. 9.4 Prone (barium in body and pylorus).

Fig. 9.5 Erect (straight-line barium-air level). Barium = white Air = black

Large Intestine

The ascending and descending portions are located more posteriorly, and thus more of these parts would be filled with barium (white) in the **supine position** and with air (black) in the **prone position.**

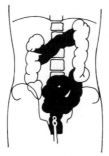

Fig. 9.6 Supine.

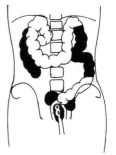

Fig. 9.7 Prone.

Note: This much separation of barium and air occurs generally only with double-contrast barium-air studies.

Air-fluid levels would be seen in the **erect position,** in which the air would rise to the highest position in each of the various sections of the large intestine, as shown in the accompanying figure.

Right and left decubitus projections (not shown on these drawings) also would demonstrate air-fluid levels, with air again rising to the highest portions.

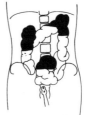

Fig. 9.8 Erect.

Acute Abdomen Series

Three-way abdomen:
- AP supine (KUB)
- AP erect
- PA chest

Two-way abdomen:
- AP supine (KUB)
- Left lateral decubitus

AP Supine (KUB): Abdomen (Adult)

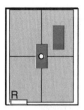

- 35 × 43 cm (14 × 17") portrait
- Grid

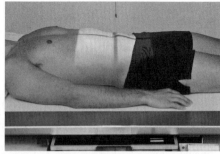

Fig. 9.9 KUB abdomen.

Position

- Supine, legs extended, arms at sides
- Midsagittal plane aligned and centered to midline of table and/or IR
- Ensure no rotation (ASISs equal distance from tabletop)
- Center of IR to level of iliac crests, ensuring that upper margin of symphysis pubis is included on lower IR margin (A large hypersthenic patient may require that the IR be placed landscape with a second IR centered higher)

Central Ray: CR ⊥, to center of IR (level of iliac crests)

SID: 40" (102 cm)

Collimation: Collimate to upper and lower abdomen soft tissue borders

Respiration: Expose at end of expiration

---

kV Range: Analog: 70–80 kV   Digital Systems:* 80 ± 5 kV

*Recommended kV ranges are similar for analog and digital systems to prevent overpenetration of small calculi in the abdomen.

	cm	kV	mA	Time	mAs	SID	Exposure Indicator
S							
M							
L							

AP Erect: Abdomen

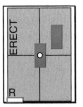

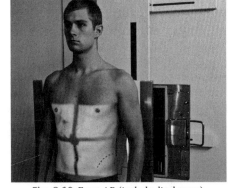

Fig. 9.10 Erect AP (include diaphragm).

- 35 × 43 cm (14 × 17″) portrait
- Grid
- Erect marker
- Patient should be on side **a minimum of 5 minutes** before exposure; a period of **10–20 minutes is preferred**

Position

- Erect, back against table, arms at sides
- Midsagittal plane aligned and centered to centerline
- Ensure no rotation
- Center of IR ≈2″ (5 cm) above iliac crest to include diaphragm (For sthenic patient, top of IR is at level of axilla)

Central Ray: CR horizontal, to center of IR (2″ [5 cm] above iliac crest)

SID: 40″ (102 cm)

Collimation: To soft tissue margins of abdomen and diaphragm

Respiration: Expose at end of expiration

kV Range:	Analog: 70–80 kV			Digital Systems: 80 ± 5 kV		

	cm	kV	mA	Time	mAs	SID	Exposure Indicator
S							
M							
L							

Abdomen and Common Contrast Media Procedures

9

Evaluation Criteria
Anatomy Demonstrated

- **AP supine:** Outline of liver, spleen, psoas muscles, and kidneys to include symphysis pubis lower abdomen
- **AP erect:** Hemidiaphragms and significant portion of lower abdomen

Position

- **AP supine and erect:** No rotation; symmetry of iliac wings and outer, lower rib margins

Exposure

- Optimal density (brightness) and contrast to visualize psoas muscles and lumbar transverse processes
- Air-fluid levels seen, if present
- Liver margins and kidneys visible on patients of average size; no motion

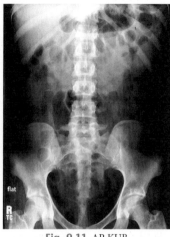

Fig. 9.11 AP KUB.

Competency Check: _____
                    Technologist   Date

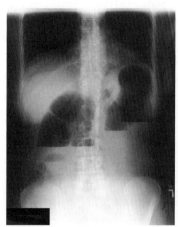

Fig. 9.12 AP erect.

Competency Check: _____
                    Technologist   Date

Lateral Decubitus (AP): Abdomen

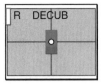

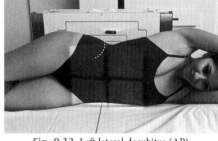

- 35 × 43 cm (14 × 17″) landscape
- Grid
- Decubitus marker
- Arrow marker to include upside

Fig. 9.13 Left lateral decubitus (AP).

- Patient should be on side **a minimum of 5 minutes** before exposure; a period of **10–20 minutes is preferred**

Position
- Lock wheels of stretcher
- Patient on side (on decubitus board or support to elevate downside abdomen), knees partially flexed, arms up near head
- Adjust patient and stretcher so that center of IR and table (and CR) is approximately 2″ (5 cm) above level of iliac crest (to include diaphragm)
- Adjust height of IR to ensure that upside of abdomen is included for possible free air

Central Ray: CR horizontal, to center of IR
SID: 40″ (102 cm)
Collimation: To soft tissue margins of abdomen and diaphragm
Respiration: Expose at end of expiration

---

kV Range: Analog: 70–80 kV   Digital Systems: 80 ± 5 kV

	cm	kV	mA	Time	mAs	SID	Exposure Indicator
S							
M							
L							

Dorsal Decubitus (Lateral): Abdomen

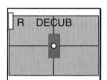

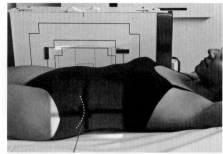

Fig. 9.14 Dorsal decubitus (R lateral).

- 35 × 43 cm (14 × 17″) landscape
- Grid
- Include decubitus marker

Abdomen and Common Contrast Media Procedures

Position

- Patient supine (on decubitus board or support to elevate posterior abdomen), side against table, arms above head
- Secure stretcher (lock wheels)
- Center of IR and table (and CR) at level of iliac crest (2″ [5 cm] above iliac crest to include diaphragm)
- Adjust height of IR to align midcoronal plane to centerline of IR

Central Ray: CR horizontal, to center of IR

SID: 40″ (102 cm)

Collimation: Collimate to upper and lower abdomen soft tissue borders

Respiration: Expose at end of expiration

kV Range:		Analog: 70–80 kV			Digital Systems: 80 ± 5 kV	
	cm	kV	mA	Time	mAs	SID	Exposure Indicator
S							
M							
L							

Bontrager Textbook, 9th ed, p. 123.

Lateral and Dorsal Decubitus: Abdomen

Evaluation Criteria
Anatomy Demonstrated

- **Lateral decubitus:** Abdomen visualized to include air-filled stomach and bowel and upside diaphragm
- **Dorsal decubitus:** Abdomen visualized to include hemidiaphragms

Position

- **Lateral decubitus: No rotation;** symmetry of iliac wings and spine straight
- **Dorsal decubitus: No rotation;** symmetry of iliac wings and diaphragm. Intervertebral joint spaces and vertebral bodies should be visible

Exposure

- Optimal density (brightness) and contrast to visualize soft tissue structures and lumbar spine
- Soft tissue structures and any intraperitoneal air demonstrated on patients of average size; no motion

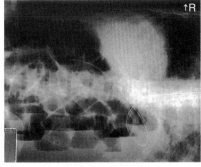

Fig. 9.15 Lateral decubitus.

Competency Check: _____
Technologist   Date

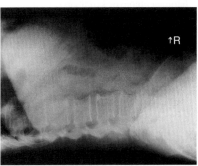

Fig. 9.16 Dorsal decubitus.

Competency Check: _____
Technologist   Date

9

AP Supine (KUB): Abdomen (Pediatric)

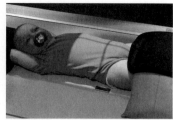

Fig. 9.17 Child AP abdomen (KUB).

- 18 × 24 cm (8 × 10″),
  24 × 30 cm (10 × 12″), or
  30 × 35 cm (11 × 14″) portrait
  (or determined by size of
  patient)
- Screen <10 cm, grid >10 cm

Position (Infant)
- Supine, immobilize arms above head (use stockinette, Ace bandage, tape, or sandbags)
- Immobilize legs with Ace bandage or tape and sandbags
- Center IR to CR
- Shield gonads, if possible

Parental Assistance for Infant: Use only if necessary. Supply with lead apron and gloves, and have parent hold patient's arms above head with one hand and legs with other hand, preventing rotation

Central Ray: *Newborns to 1 year old:* CR to 1″ (2.5 cm) above umbilicus. *Older child:* CR to level of iliac crest

SID: 40″ (102 cm)

Collimation: On four sides to abdominal borders

Respiration: Expose on expiration or when abdomen has least movement. If crying, time exposures at full expiration

kV Range:	Analog: 65–75 kV			Digital Systems: 70–80 kV		
	cm	kV	mA	Time	mAs	SID	Exposure Indicator
S							
M							
L							

Bontrager Textbook, 9th ed, p. 640.

AP Erect: Abdomen (Pediatric)

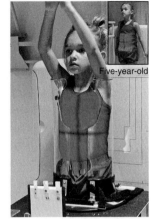

Fig. 9.18 Utilizing Pigg-O-Stat.

- 18 × 24 cm (8 × 10″), 24 × 30 cm (10 × 12″), or 30 × 35 cm (11 × 14″) portrait (or determined by size of patient)
- Screen <10 cm, grid >10 cm

Position
- Patient seated, legs through openings
- Arms above head, side body clamps firmly in place
- Lead shield at level of symphysis pubis; center IR to CR

Parental Assistance: If necessary, have parent hold arms overhead with one hand, and with other hand hold legs to prevent rotation of pelvis or thorax (provide with lead apron and gloves)

Central Ray: *Newborn–1 year old:* CR to 1″ (2.5 cm) above umbilicus. *Older child:* CR ≈1–2″ (2.5–5 cm) (depending on the height of the child) above the level of the iliac crest

SID: 40″ (102 cm)

Collimation: On four sides to abdominal borders

Respiration: Expose on expiration, or during least movement

---

kV Range:		Analog: 65–75 kV		Digital Systems: 70–85 kV			
	cm	kV	mA	Time	mAs	SID	Exposure Indicator
S							
M							
L							

AP Supine and Erect: Abdomen (Pediatric)

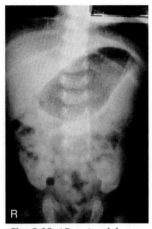

Fig. 9.19 AP supine abdomen.

Competency Check: _____
                    Technologist   Date

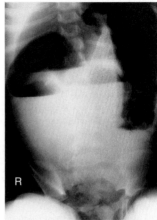

Fig. 9.20 Erect AP abdomen.

Competency Check: _____
                    Technologist   Date

Evaluation Criteria

Anatomy Demonstrated

- **AP supine and erect:** Soft tissue and gas-filled structures; air-fluid levels on erect

Position

- **AP supine and erect:** Diaphragm to symphysis pubis included, if possible

Exposure

- Optimal density (brightness) and contrast to visualize soft tissue structures and skeletal structures; no motion

9

RAO: Esophagogram

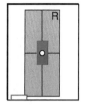

- 35 × 43 cm (14 × 17″) portrait
- Grid

Position
- Recumbent or erect, recumbent preferred for more complete filling of esophagus
- Rotate 35°–40° from prone position onto right side, right arm down, left arm up; hold cup with left hand, straw in mouth
- Center thorax to centerline
- Top of IR ≈2″ (5 cm) above level of shoulder

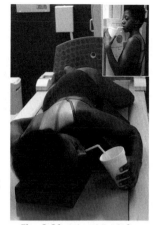

Fig. 9.21 35°–40° RAO for esophagus (barium swallow).

Central Ray: CR ⊥, to center of IR (≈2–3″ [5–8 cm] inferior to jugular notch at T6 level)

SID: 40″ (102 cm)

Collimation: To area of interest (≈5–6″ [12–15 cm] wide)

Respiration: With thin barium, expose while swallowing (after 3 or 4 swallows). With thick barium, expose immediately after swallowing. The patient generally does not breathe immediately after a swallow.

	cm	kV	mA	Time	mAs	SID	Exposure Indicator
kV Range:			Analog and Digital Systems: 110–125 kV				
S							
M							
L							

Abdomen and Common Contrast Media Procedures

9

Lateral: Esophagogram

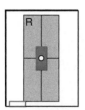

- 35 × 43 cm (14 × 17") portrait
- Grid

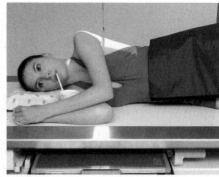

Fig. 9.22 R lateral esophagogram (barium swallow).

Position
- Recumbent or erect; recumbent preferred
- Right lateral position, right arm and shoulder up and forward (holding cup)
- Center midcoronal plane to centerline
- Top of IR ≈2" (5 cm) above top of shoulder

Central Ray: CR ⊥, to center of IR (≈2–3" [5–8 cm] inferior to jugular notch at T6 level)

SID: 40" (102 cm) or 72" (183 cm) if performed erect

Collimation: To area of interest (5–6" [12–15 cm] wide)

Respiration: With thin barium, expose while patient is swallowing (after 3 or 4 swallows). With thick barium, expose immediately after patient swallows. The patient generally does not breathe immediately after a swallow.

kV Range:				Analog and Digital Systems: 110–125 kV		
	cm	kV	mA	Time	mAs	SID	Exposure Indicator
S							
M							
L							

Bontrager Textbook, 9th ed, p. 479.

RAO and Lateral: Esophagogram

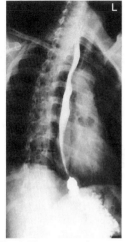

Fig. 9.23 RAO esophagogram.

Competency Check: _____
Technologist   Date

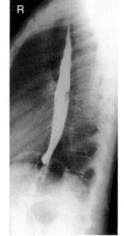

Fig. 9.24 Right lateral esophagogram.

Competency Check: _____
Technologist   Date

Evaluation Criteria

Anatomy Demonstrated

- **RAO:** Esophagus visible between vertebral column and heart
- **Lateral:** Entire esophagus visible between thoracic spine and heart

Position

- **RAO:** Entire esophagus lined with contrast media and not superimposed over spine
- **Lateral:** No rotation; superimposition of posterior ribs, entire esophagus lined with contrast media

Exposure

- Optimal density (brightness) and contrast to visualize borders of contrast-filled esophagus
- Sharp structural margins; no motion

Abdomen and Common Contrast Media Procedures

9

285

AP (PA): Esophagogram

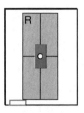

- 35 × 43 cm (14 × 17″) portrait
- Grid

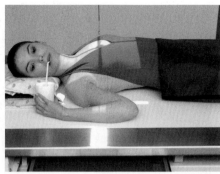

Fig. 9.25 AP esophagogram (barium swallow).

Position

- Supine or erect;
  supine preferred (may be performed PA if erect)
- Center patient to midline of table
- Top of IR ≈2″ (5 cm) above top of shoulder
- Left arm at side, holding cup with right hand, straw in mouth

Central Ray: CR ⊥, to center of IR (≈3″ [8 cm] inferior to jugular notch at T6)

SID: 40″ (102 cm) or 72″ (183 cm) if performed erect

Collimation: To area of interest (5–6″ [12–15 cm] wide)

Respiration: With thin barium, expose while patient is swallowing (after 3 or 4 swallows). With thick barium, expose immediately after patient swallows

kV Range:				Analog and Digital Systems: **110–125 kV**		
	cm	kV	mA	Time	mAs	SID	Exposure Indicator
S							
M							
L							

Bontrager Textbook, 9th ed., p. 480.

PA: Upper GI (Stomach)

- 35 × 43 cm (14 × 17″), 30 × 35 cm (11 × 14″), or 24 × 30 cm (10 × 12″) portrait
- Grid

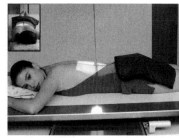

Fig. 9.26 PA upper GI (stomach).

Position
- Prone, arms up beside head
- Align and center patient and IR to CR

Central Ray: CR ⊥, centered as follows:

Sthenic: Center ≈1–2″ (2.5–5 cm) above lower rib margin (level of L1) and ≈1″ (2.5 cm) to left of vertebral column

Hypersthenic: Center 2″ (5 cm) above level of L1 nearer midline

Asthenic: Center ≈2″ (5 cm) below level of T1 and nearer midline

SID: 40″ (102 cm)

Collimation: To outer margins of IR or to area of interest

Respiration: Expose at end of expiration

Abdomen and Common Contrast Media Procedures

kV Range:		Analog and Digital Systems: 110–125 kV
		90–100 kV (Double-Contrast)
		80–90 kV (Water-Soluble Contrast Media)

	cm	kV	mA	Time	mAs	SID	Exposure Indicator
S							
M							
L							

9

RAO: Upper GI (Stomach)

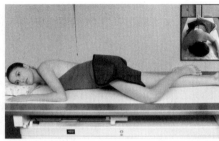

Fig. 9.27 40°–70° RAO, upper GI (stomach).

- 30 × 35 cm (11 × 14″) or 24 × 30 cm (10 × 12″) portrait
- Grid

Position

- Semiprone, rotate 40°–70° from prone with right anterior side against table
- Right arm down, left arm up, partially flex left hip and knee
- Align and center patient to CR

Central Ray: CR ⊥ to IR

Sthenic: Center ≈1–2″ (2.5–5 cm) above lower ribs and midway between spine and upside left lateral abdominal border, 45°–55° oblique from prone

Hypersthenic: Center 2″ (5 cm) above level of L1 and nearer midline, ≈70° oblique

Asthenic: Center ≈2″ (5 cm) below level of L1, ≈40° oblique

SID: 40″ (102 cm)

Collimation: To outer margins of IR or to area of interest

Respiration: Expose at end of expiration

kV Range:			Analog and Digital Systems: 110–125 kV
			90–100 kV (Double-Contrast)
			80–90 kV (Water-Soluble Contrast Media)

	cm	kV	mA	Time	mAs	SID	Exposure Indicator
S							
M							
L							

Bontrager Textbook, 9th ed, p. 482.

PA and RAO: Upper GI (Stomach)

Evaluation Criteria
Anatomy Demonstrated
- **PA:** Entire stomach and duodenum
- **RAO:** Entire stomach and C-loop of duodenum

Position
- **PA:** Body and pylorus are barium-filled; body and pylorus are centered
- **RAO:** Pylorus and duodenal bulb in profile and barium-filled

Exposure
- Optimal density (brightness) and contrast to visualize gastric folds without overexposing other structures
- Sharp structural margins; no motion

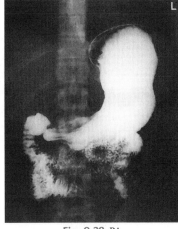

Fig. 9.28 PA.

Competency Check: _____
  Technologist   Date

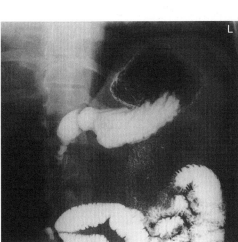

Fig. 9.29 RAO.

Competency Check: _____
  Technologist   Date

Right Lateral: Upper GI (Stomach)

- 30 × 35 cm (11 × 14") or 24 × 30 cm (10 × 12") portrait
- Grid

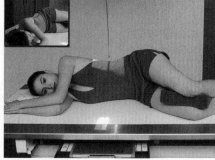

Fig. 9.30 Right lateral upper GI (stomach).

Position
- Patient on right side, arms up, hips and knees partially flexed
- Align and center patient and IR to CR

Central Ray: CR ⊥ to the IR

Sthenic: Center to margin of ribs at level of L1, and 1–1½″ (2.5–4 cm) anterior to midcoronal plane (near midway between anterior border of vertebrae and anterior abdomen)

Hypersthenic: Center ≈2″ (5 cm) above L1

Asthenic: Center ≈2″ (5 cm) below L1

SID: 40″ (102 cm)

Collimation: To outer margins of IR or to area of interest

Respiration: Expose at end of expiration

---

kV Range:	Analog and Digital Systems: 110–125 kV
	90–100 kV (Double-Contrast)
	80–90 kV (Water-Soluble Contrast Media)

	cm	kV	mA	Time	mAs	SID	Exposure Indicator
S							
M							
L							

Bontrager Textbook, 9th ed, p. 484.

AP: Upper GI (Stomach)

- 30 × 35 cm (11 × 14″) or 35 × 43 cm (14 × 17″) portrait
- Grid

Position

- Supine, arms at side
- Align and center patient and IR to CR

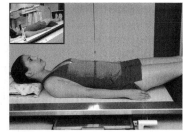

Fig. 9.31 AP supine Trendelenburg, upper GI (stomach) (Trendelenburg position best demonstrates hiatal hernia).

Central Ray: CR ⊥ to IR, centered to 2.5–5 cm (1–2″) to left of MSP

Sthenic: Center to level of L1 (midway between xiphoid process and level of lower lateral ribs)

Hypersthenic: Center ≈5 cm (2″) above level of L1

Asthenic: Center ≈5 cm (2″) below level of L1 and nearer midline

SID: 40″ (102 cm)

Collimation: To outer IR margins or to area of interest

Respiration: Expose at end of expiration

kV Range:	Analog and Digital Systems: 110–125 kV
	90–100 kV (Double-Contrast)
	80–90 kV (Water-Soluble Contrast Media)

	cm	kV	mA	Time	mAs	SID	Exposure Indicator
S							
M							
L							

Abdomen and Common Contrast Media Procedures

9

Abdomen and Common Contrast Media Procedures

9

Evaluation Criteria

Anatomy Demonstrated

- **Right lateral:** Entire stomach and duodenum and retrogastric space demonstrated
- **AP:** Entire stomach and C-loop of duodenum; diaphragm included to r/o hiatal hernia

Position

- **Right lateral:** Pylorus and C-loop of duodenum demonstrated. **No rotation;** evident by aligned vertebral bodies
- **AP:** Fundus barium-filled and centered

Exposure

- Optimal density (brightness) and contrast to visualize gastric folds without overexposing other structures
- Sharp structural margins; no motion

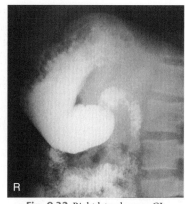

Fig. 9.32 Right lateral upper GI.

Competency Check: _____
                   Technologist   Date

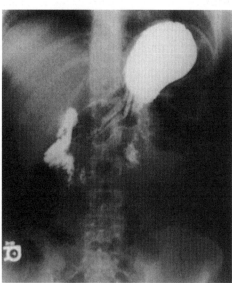

Fig. 9.33 AP upper GI.

Competency Check: _____
                   Technologist   Date

LPO: Upper GI (Stomach)

- 30 × 35 cm (11 × 14″) or 24 × 30 cm (10 × 12″) portrait
- Grid

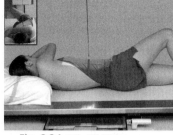

Fig. 9.34 30°–60° LPO, upper GI (stomach).

Position

- Semisupine, 30°–60° oblique,* left side down, partially flex right knee
- Center patient and IR to CR

*Up to 60° for hypersthenic patients and 30° for asthenic patients

Central Ray: CR ⊥ to IR, centered to left half of abdomen

Sthenic: Center to L1 (midway between xiphoid process and level of lower lateral ribs), 45° oblique

Hypersthenic: Center 5 cm (2″) above L1, 60° oblique

Asthenic: ≈5 cm (2″) below L1 and nearer midline, 30° oblique

SID: 40″ (102 cm)

Collimation: To outer IR margins or to area of interest

Respiration: Expose at end of expiration

kV Range: Analog and Digital Systems: 110–125 kV
                           90–100 kV (Double-Contrast)
                   80–90 kV (Water-Soluble Contrast Media)

	cm	kV	mA	Time	mAs	SID	Exposure Indicator
S							
M							
L							

Abdomen and Common Contrast Media Procedures

9

LPO: Upper GI (Stomach)

Evaluation Criteria
Anatomy Demonstrated
- Entire stomach and duodenum; unobstructed view of duodenal bulb

Position
- Fundus is barium-filled; gas-filled duodenal bulb seen for double-contrast study
- Duodenal bulb in profile

Exposure
- Optimal density (brightness) and contrast to visualize gastric folds without overexposing other structures
- Sharp structural and gastric organ margins; no motion

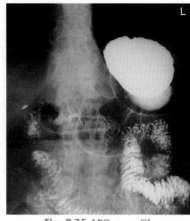

Fig. 9.35 LPO upper GI.

Competency Check: _____

Technologist   Date

PA: Small Bowel

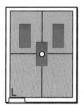

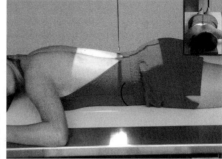

A common routine includes images at 15- or 30-minute intervals until barium reaches ileocecal valve.

Fig. 9.36 PA small bowel (15 or 30 minutes).

- 35 × 43 cm (14 × 17″) portrait
- Grid
- Time indicators visible on image

Position

- Prone preferred (may be taken AP supine, if necessary)
- MSP aligned to midline of table; no rotation
- Center patient and IR to iliac crest (center higher on early IRs)

Central Ray: CR ⊥ to IR, to center of IR, ≈2″ (5 cm) above level of iliac crest for early IRs (15 or 30 minutes), and at iliac crest for later images

SID: 40″ (102 cm)

Collimation: To outer margins of IR or to area of interest

Respiration: Expose at end of full expiration

Note: Imaging series and technical factors are similar for enteroclysis and intubation procedures

kV Range:		Analog and Digital Systems: 110–125 kV				
	cm	kV	mA	Time	mAs	SID	Exposure Indicator
S							
M							
L							

Abdomen and Common Contrast Media Procedures

9

PA (AP): Barium Enema

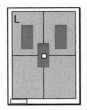

- 35 × 43 cm
  (14 × 17″) portrait
- Grid

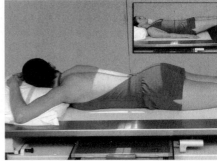

Fig. 9.37 PA barium enema.

Position
- Patient prone (PA)
  or supine (AP)
- Patient aligned and centered to centerline; no rotation
- Center IR to level of iliac crest (see *Note*)

Central Ray: CR ⊥ to IR, to center of IR, at level of iliac crest

Note: For large or hypersthenic patients, the use of two IRs may be necessary, placed landscape if the entire large intestine is to be included (one centered for lower abdomen and one for upper abdomen)

SID: 40″ (102 cm)

Collimation: To outer IR borders or to area of interest

Respiration: Expose at full expiration

kV Range:				Analog and Digital Systems:			
				110–125 kV (Single Contrast)			
				90–100 kV (Double Contrast)			
				80–90 kV (Water-Soluble Contrast Media)			

	cm	kV	mA	Time	mAs	SID	Exposure Indicator
S							
M							
L							

Bontrager Textbook, 9th ed, p. 515.

Evaluation Criteria

Anatomy Demonstrated

- Entire large intestine demonstrated, including left colic flexure and rectum

Position

- Transverse colon primarily filled with barium (PA) and gas-filled with AP
- **No rotation;** evident by symmetry of ala of ilium and lumbar vertebra

Exposure

- Optimal density (brightness) and contrast to visualize mucosa without overexposing other structures
- Sharp structural margins; no motion

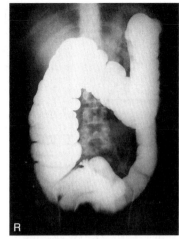

Fig. 9.38 PA single-contrast BE.

Competency Check: _____
                   Technologist   Date

Abdomen and Common Contrast Media Procedures

9

RAO and LAO (RPO and LPO): Barium Enema

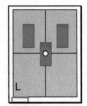

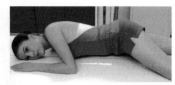

Fig. 9.39 35°–45° RAO barium enema.

Both right and left oblique projections are commonly performed.
- 35 × 43 cm (14 × 17″) portrait
- Grid

Position
- Semiprone (PA) or semisupine (AP), rotated 35°–45°
- Align and center abdomen to midline of table.
- IR centered to level of iliac crest (include rectal area)

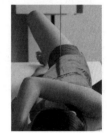

Fig. 9.40 35°–45° LPO.

Central Ray: CR ⊥ to center of IR (at level 1–2″ [2.5–5 cm] above iliac crest) ≈1″ (2.5 cm) to the left of the MSP

Note: Many patients require a second IR centered ≈2″ (5 cm) higher if the left colic flexure is to be included—most important on LAO or RPO (determine departmental routine).

SID: 40″ (102 cm)

Collimation: To outer IR borders or to area of interest

Respiration: Expose at expiration

kV Range:				Analog and Digital Systems:			
				110–125 kV (Single Contrast)			
				90–100 kV (Double Contrast)			
				80–90 kV (Water-Soluble Contrast Media)			
	cm	kV	mA	Time	mAs	SID	Exposure Indicator
S							
M							
L							

Bontrager Textbook, 9th ed, pp. 516 and 517.

RAO and LAO (RPO and LPO): Barium Enema

Evaluation Criteria

Anatomy Demonstrated
- **LPO/RAO:** Right colic flexure and ascending and sigmoid colon
- **RPO/LAO:** Left colic flexure and descending colon

Position
- **LPO/RAO:** Right colic flexure and ascending colon in profile
- **RPO/LAO:** Left colic flexure in profile and descending colon in profile

Exposure
- Appropriate technique (brightness) to visualize mucosa without overexposing other structures
- Sharp structural margins; no motion

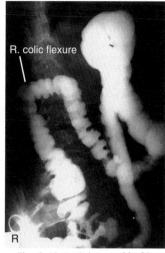

R. colic flexure

R

Fig. 9.41 RAO (centered high).

Competency Check: _____

Technologist   Date

L. colic flexure

Fig. 9.42 RPO.

Competency Check: _____

Technologist   Date

Lateral Rectum (Ventral Decubitus): Barium Enema

Alternative ventral decubitus projection is often performed for double-contrast studies.

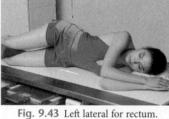

Fig. 9.43 Left lateral for rectum.

- 30 × 35 cm (11 × 14″) or 24 × 30 cm (10 × 12″) portrait
- Grid
- Compensating filter for ventral decubitus lateral recommended

Position

- Recumbent in true lateral position
- Center midaxillary plane to midline of table, with knees and hips partially flexed
- Center patient and IR to CR

Fig. 9.44 Ventral decubitus lateral rectum (alternate projection with double-contrast examination).

Central Ray: CR ⊥ to IR, to level of ASIS, centered to midcoronal plane (midway between ASIS and posterior sacrum). CR is horizontal for ventral decubitus

SID: 40″ (102 cm)

Collimation: To outer IR borders or to area of interest

Respiration: Expose at expiration

---

kV Range: Analog and Digital Systems:

110–125 kV (Single Contrast) 90–100 kV (Double Contrast)
80–90 kV (Water-Soluble Contrast Media)

	cm	kV	mA	Time	mAs	SID	Exposure Indicator
S							
M							
L							

300 Bontrager Textbook, 9th ed, p. 519.

Lateral Decubitus (Double Contrast): Barium Enema

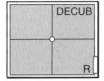

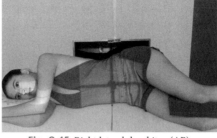

Fig. 9.45 Right lateral decubitus (AP).

Both right and left lateral decubitus are commonly performed as part of a double-contrast series.

- 35 × 43 cm (14 × 17″) portrait to patient
- Grid (portable grid or bucky)
- Compensating filter placed on upside of abdomen

Position

- Patient on side, arms up, knees partially flexed, back against grid cassette or table
- MSP aligned and centered to centerline of IR (and CR); no rotation (lock wheels if stretcher is used)
- IR centered to level of iliac crest

Central Ray: CR horizontal to center of IR (to level of iliac crest at midsagittal plane)

SID: 40″ (102 cm)

Collimation: To outer IR borders or to area of interest

Respiration: Expose at full expiration

---

kV Range:		Analog and Digital Systems: 90–100 kV (Double-Contrast Study)				

	cm	kV	mA	Time	mAs	SID	Exposure Indicator
S							
M							
L							

Bontrager Textbook, 9th ed, p. 520.

AP (PA) Axial: Barium Enema

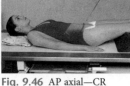

Fig. 9.46 AP axial—CR 30°–45° cephalad.

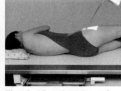

Fig. 9.47 35° LPO axial—CR 30°–40° cephalad.

- 30 × 35 cm (11 × 14″) portrait
- Grid

Position
Supine (AP) or Prone (PA): Patient aligned and centered to centerline
Alternate Oblique: LPO or RAO: Oblique patient 30°–40°
Central Ray: CR 30°–40° cephalad for AP; 30°–40° caudad for PA
AP axial: CR to 2″ (5 cm) inferior to ASIS
PA axial: CR to enter at level of ASIS
LPO axial: CR 2″ (5 cm) inferior and 2″ (5 cm) medial to right ASIS
SID: 40″ (102 cm)
Collimation: To area of interest
Respiration: Expose at full expiration

kV Range:				Analog and Digital Systems:		
				110–125 kV (Single Contrast)		
				90–100 kV (Double Contrast)		
				80–90 kV (Water-Soluble Contrast Media)		

	cm	kV	mA	Time	mAs	SID	Exposure Indicator
S							
M							
L							

Bontrager Textbook, 9th ed, p. 523.

Lateral Decubitus and AP (PA) Axial: Barium Enema

Evaluation Criteria

Anatomy Demonstrated

- **Lateral decubitus:** Entire large intestine demonstrated
- **AP/PA axial:** Elongated views of rectosigmoid colon

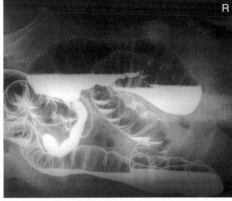

Fig. 9.48 Left lateral decubitus.

Competency Check: _____
　　　　　　　　　Technologist　　　　　　　Date

Position

- **Lateral decubitus: No rotation** evident by symmetry of pelvis and ribs
- **AP/PA axial:** Less superimposition between rectum and sigmoid colon

Exposure

- Appropriate technique (brightness) to visualize mucosa without overexposing other structures
- Sharp structural margins; no motion

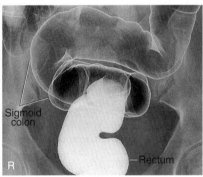

Sigmoid colon

Rectum

Fig. 9.49 AP axial.

Competency Check: _____
　　　　　　　　　Technologist　　　　　　　Date

9

AP (PA) Scout and Series: Intravenous Urogram (IVU)

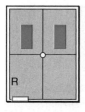

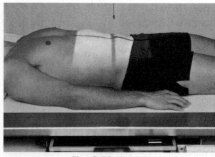

Fig. 9.50 AP IVU.

- 35 × 43 cm (14 × 17″) portrait; 30 × 35 cm (11 × 14″) for nephrotomography, landscape
- Grid
- Include minute markers, where applicable
- Note that early images may include nephrotomography
- Shield gonads for males

Position

- Supine, midsagittal plane aligned and centered to midline of table; support placed under knees; no rotation

Central Ray: CR ⊥, to center of IR, at level of iliac crest, or 1–2″ (2.5–5 cm) above crests on long-torso patients with second smaller IR landscape for bladder area, to include symphysis pubis on lower border of IR. *Nephrography:* Center CR midway between xiphoid process and iliac crest.

SID: 40″ (102 cm)

Collimation: To outer margins of IR or area of interest

Respiration: Expose at end of full expiration

kV Range:	Analog: 70–75 kV				Digital Systems: 80 ± 5 kV	
	cm	kV	mA	Time	mAs	SID	Exposure Indicator
S							
M							
L							

RPO and LPO: IVU

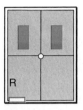

Both R and L posterior oblique projections should be part of routine.

- 35 × 43 cm (14 × 17″) portrait
- Grid
- Include minute marker
- Shield gonads for males

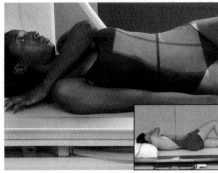

Fig. 9.51 30°—RPO (*Insert:* LPO).

Position
- Semisupine, 30° oblique to right (or left), flex elevated knee and elbow, as shown, for support (place angled support under back, if needed)
- Align and center abdomen to centerline
- Center IR to level of iliac crest

Central Ray: CR ⊥, to center of IR, at level of iliac crest
SID: 40″ (102 cm)
Collimation: To outer margins of IR or to area of interest
Respiration: Expose at end of full expiration

| kV Range: | Analog: 70–75 kV | | | | Digital Systems: 80 ± 5 kV | |

	cm	kV	mA	Time	mAs	SID	Exposure Indicator
S							
M							
L							

Abdomen and Common Contrast Media Procedures

9

Evaluation Criteria
Anatomy Demonstrated
- **AP and oblique:** Entire urinary system visualized from renal shadows to symphysis pubis

Position
- **AP:** No rotation; evident by symmetry of iliac wings; symphysis pubis and top of kidneys included
- **Oblique:** Kidney on elevated side in profile; downside ureter away from spine

Exposure
- Appropriate technique (brightness) and contrast to visualize kidneys and ureters without overexposing other structures; no motion
- Minute and side markers visible

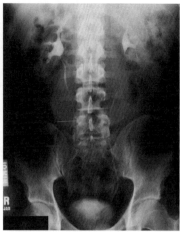

Fig. 9.52 AP—10 minutes (postinjection).

Competency Check: _____

                    Technologist   Date

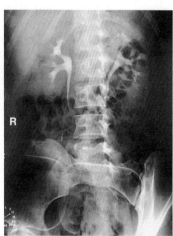

Fig. 9.53 30°—RPO. (From Frank ED, Long BW, Smith BJ: Merrill's atlas of radiographic positioning and procedures, ed 12, St. Louis, 2012, Elsevier.)

Competency Check: _____

                    Technologist   Date

AP Erect (Postvoid): IVU

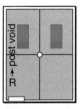

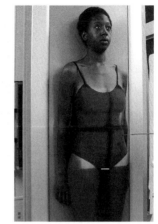

Fig. 9.54 AP erect postvoid.

- 35 × 43 cm (14 × 17″) portrait
- Grid
- Erect and postvoid markers

Position
- Erect, midsagittal plane aligned and centered to midline of table, no rotation
- Center IR to iliac crest—ensure that bladder area, including the symphysis pubis

Central Ray: CR ⊥, to center of IR (at level of iliac crests or ≈1″ [2.5 cm] lower than crest to include bladder area)

SID: 40″ (102 cm)

Collimation: To outer margins of IR or to area of interest

Respiration: Expose at end of full expiration

kV Range:		Analog: 70–75 kV			Digital Systems: 80 ± 5 kV		
	cm	kV	mA	Time	mAs	SID	Exposure Indicator
S							
M							
L							

Bontrager Textbook, 9th ed, p. 557.

AP Axial: Cystography

R

- 30 × 35 cm (11 × 14″) portrait for adult
- Grid

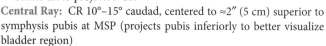

Fig. 9.55 AP axial—CR 10°–15° caudad.

Position

- Supine, midsagittal plane aligned and centered to midline of table, legs fully extended
- Center IR to projected CR

Central Ray: CR 10°–15° caudad, centered to ≈2″ (5 cm) superior to symphysis pubis at MSP (projects pubis inferiorly to better visualize bladder region)

SID: 40″ (102 cm)

Collimation: To outer margins of IR or area of interest

Respiration: Expose at end of full expiration

kV Range:		Analog: 70–75 kV				Digital Systems: 80 ± 5 kV	
	cm	kV	mA	Time	mAs	SID	Exposure Indicator
S							
M							
L							

Bontrager Textbook, 9th ed, p. 559.

Posterior Oblique (RPO, LPO) and Optional Lateral: Cystography

Note: Cystogram routine may not include a lateral because of high gonadal dose.

- 30 × 35 cm (11 × 14″) portrait
- Grid

Position

- Semisupine, 45°–60° oblique (60° oblique best demonstrates posterolateral bladder and UV junction)
- Flex elevated arm and leg to support this position
- Center patient and IR to CR

Central Ray: CR ⊥ to IR, to ≈2″ (5 cm) superior to symphysis pubis, and 2″ (5 cm) medial to elevated ASIS

SID: 40″ (102 cm)

Collimation: To margins of IR or area of interest

Respiration: Expose at expiration

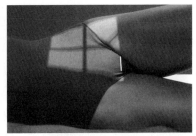

Fig. 9.56 45° RPO.

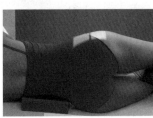

Fig. 9.57 Optional lateral. —CR ⊥, 2″ (5 cm) superior and post to symphysis pubis.

kV Range:	AP Oblique—Analog: 70–75 kV
	Digital Systems: 80–85 kV
	Lateral—Analog and Digital Systems: 80 ± 5 kV

	cm	kV	mA	Time	mAs	SID	Exposure Indicator
S							
M							
L							

Abdomen and Common Contrast Media Procedures

9

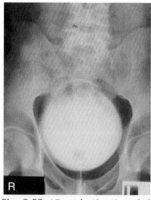

Fig. 9.58 AP axial 10°–15° caudad.

Competency Check: _____
　　　　　　　　　Technologist　　Date

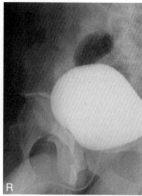

Fig. 9.59 45° posterior oblique.

Competency Check: _____
　　　　　　　　　Technologist　　Date

Abdomen and Common Contrast Media Procedures

Evaluation Criteria

Anatomy Demonstrated

- **AP axial and Oblique:** Distal ureters, bladder, and proximal urethra

Position

- **AP axial:** Urinary bladder not superimposed by pubic bones
- **Oblique:** Urinary bladder not superimposed by partially flexed leg

Exposure

- Appropriate technique (brightness) to visualize urinary bladder without overexposing other structures; no motion

9

Chapter 10

Mobile (Portables) and Surgical Procedures

Essential Principles for Trauma and Mobile Radiography

The following three principles must be observed for trauma and mobile procedures:

- **Two projections 90° to each other (minimum):** Trauma radiography generally requires two projections taken at 90° (or right angles to each other) while true CR-part-IR alignment is maintained.
- **Entire anatomic structure or trauma area on image receptor:** Trauma radiography mandates that the entire structure being examined should be included on the radiographic image to ensure that no pathologic condition is missed. Additional projections must be performed if the entire structure is not seen on the initial image.
- **Maintain the safety of the patient, health care workers, and the public:** Technologists must maintain the safety and well-being of patients, family/friends, and other health care workers during a trauma or mobile radiographic procedure. Safe handling of patients and radiation protection of the patient and others in the immediate vicinity of the exposure is the responsibility of the technologist.

Shielding
- Shield all radiosensitive tissues outside the region of interest, when appropriate, during mobile imaging series.

311

AP Chest (Supine and Semierect): Mobile

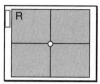

- 35 × 43 cm (14 × 17″) landscape or portrait
- Nongrid or grid

Position
- Cover IR with plastic case, center to patient with top of IR approximately 2″ (5 cm) above shoulders
- Supine, elevate head end of bed, if possible, into seated or semierect position
- Ensure no rotation of patient
- If patient condition allows, rotate shoulders forward

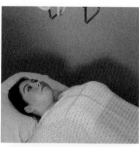

Fig. 10.1 Supine AP chest.

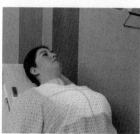

Fig. 10.2 Semierect AP chest.

Central Ray:
- CR 3°–5° caudal from perpendicular to IR so as to be perpendicular to sternum (prevents clavicles from obscuring apices of lungs)
- Center CR to 3–4″ (8–10 cm) below jugular notch at level of T7

SID: 48–72″ (123–183 cm); use greater SID, if possible

Respiration: Expose after second full inspiration

| | kV Range: | | Analog and Digital Systems: **90–125 kV*** |

*Lower kV for nongrid procedures.

	cm	kV	mA	Time	mAs	SID	Exposure Indicator
S							
M							
L							

Bontrager Textbook, 9th ed, p. 573.

AP Supine Abdomen (KUB): Mobile

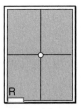

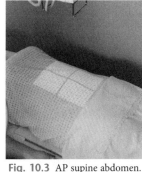

Fig. 10.3 AP supine abdomen.

- 35 × 43 cm (14 × 17″) portrait
- Grid

Position
- Cover IR with plastic case
- Center IR to patient at level of iliac crest
- Place supports under IR, if needed, to ensure IR is level and perpendicular to CR (prevents patient rotation and grid cutoff)

Central Ray: CR perpendicular to IR, centered to IR at level of iliac crest

SID: 40″ (102 cm)

Respiration: Expose on expiration

	cm	kV	mA	Time	mAs	SID	Exposure Indicator
S							
M							
L							

kV Range: Analog 70–80 kV   Digital Systems 80 ± 5 kV

10

Lateral Decubitus (Abdomen): Mobile

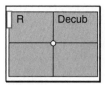

Left lateral best demonstrates free air in right upper abdomen. Must include diaphragm.

- 35 × 43 cm (14 × 17″) landscape (to anatomy)
- Grid
- Decubitus marker

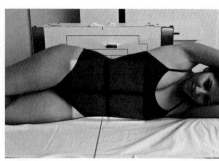

Fig. 10.4 AP left lateral decubitus abdomen.

Position

- Patient on left (or right if indicated) side with support, as shown, to prevent sinking into soft bed
- Center of IR 2″ (5 cm) above level of iliac crest to include diaphragm
- Ensure no rotation and that the IR plane is perpendicular to CR

Central Ray: Horizontal CR to center of IR 2″ (5 cm) above iliac crest
SID: 40″ (102 cm)
Respiration: Expose on expiration
Note: Have patient on side **5 minutes** (minimum) before exposure; a period of **10–20 minutes is preferred.** Ensure that diaphragm and upside of abdomen are included.

	kV Range:	Analog 70–80 kV				Digital Systems 80 ± 5 kV	
	cm	kV	mA	Time	mAs	SID	Exposure Indicator
S							
M							
L							

10

Bontrager Textbook, 9th ed., p. 575.

AP Pelvis or Hip: Mobile

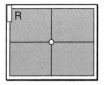

- **Pelvis:** 35 × 43 cm (14 × 17″) landscape
- **Hip only:** 24 × 30 cm (10 × 12″) portrait
- Grid

Position—Pelvis
- Cover IR with plastic case, slide IR under patient, centered landscape to patient
- Top of IR ≈1″ (2.5 cm) above iliac crest
- Ensure no rotation of patient (equal ASIS distances to IR)
- Internally rotate both legs 15° only if hip fracture is not suspected

Central Ray: CR perpendicular midway between ASIS and symphysis pubis

AP Hip: Center CR and IR to hip region (2″ [5 cm] medial to ASIS at level of greater trochanter)

SID: 40″ (102 cm)

Respiration: Suspend during exposure

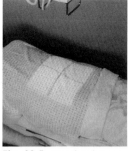

Fig. 10.5 AP pelvis (trauma hip without leg rotation).

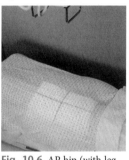

Fig. 10.6 AP hip (with leg rotation).

Mobile (Portables) and Surgical Procedures

kV Range:			Analog	Digital Systems
	Distal Femur		80 ± 5 kV	80 ± 5 kV
	Proximal Femur/Pelvis		80 ± 5 kV	85 ± 5 kV

	cm	kV	mA	Time	mAs	SID	Exposure Indicator
S							
M							
L							

10

Axiolateral Hip
(Danelius-Miller Method): Mobile

- 24 × 30 cm (10 × 12″) landscape (long axis of IR aligned to long axis of femur)
- Grid

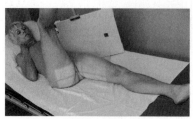

Fig. 10.7 Axiolateral hip.

Position
- Place folded towels or support under affected hip
- Place vertical grid against patient's side with top of IR at the level of the iliac crest with face of grid parallel to femoral neck and perpendicular to CR
- Elevate opposite leg (**DO NOT** support leg/foot on collimator or tube because of risk for burns or electrical shock)
- Internally rotate affected leg only if unsecured hip fracture is not suspected

Central Ray: Horizontal CR angled to be perpendicular to IR and femoral neck
SID: 40″ (102 cm)
Respiration: Suspend during exposure

kV Range:		Analog: 80 ± 5 kV			Digital Systems: 85 ± 5 kV		
	cm	kV	mA	Time	mAs	SID	Exposure Indicator
S							
M							
L							

10

Bontrager Textbook, 9th ed, p. 586.

Modified Axiolateral Hip and Proximal Femur (Clements-Nakayama Method): Mobile

Alternative projection if both limbs have limited movement and the inferosuperior projection cannot be obtained

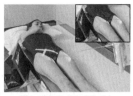

Fig. 10.8 Modified axiolateral projection.

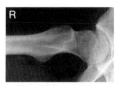

Fig. 10.9 Lateral proximal femur (modified axiolateral projection).

- 24 × 30 cm (10 × 12″) landscape
- Grid (aligned to CR angle to prevent grid cutoff)

Position

- Patient supine, affected side near edge of table with both legs fully extended
- Provide pillow for head, and place arms across superior chest
- Maintain leg in neutral (anatomical) position
- Rest IR on extended bucky tray, which places the bottom edge of the IR about 2″ (5 cm) below the level of the tabletop
- Tilt IR approximately 15° from vertical and adjust alignment of IR to ensure that face of IR is **perpendicular** to CR to prevent grid cutoff
- Center centerline of IR to projected CR

Central Ray: Angle CR **mediolaterally** as needed so that it is **perpendicular to** and **centered to femoral neck** (≈**15°–20°** posteriorly from horizontal)

SID: 40″ (102 cm)

	cm	kV	mA	Time	mAs	SID	Exposure Indicator
S							
M							
L							

kV Range: Analog: 80 ± 5 kV   Digital Systems: 85 ± 5 kV

Mobile (Portables) and Surgical Procedures

10

PA Abdomen (Cholangiogram): Surgical C-Arm

Position and CR
- PA projection (patient supine): Image intensifier on top, tube below
- Provide lead aprons or portable shields for all personnel in room
- Maintain sterile field
- Automatic or manual exposure control

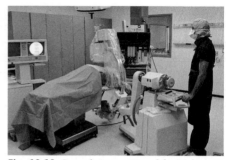

Fig. 10.10 C-arm being positioned for PA hip or abdomen.

- Foot pedal allows hands-free operation by physician of fluoroscopic image as displayed on monitor

---

Lateral Hip: Surgical C-Arm

Position and CR
- Superoinferior projection
  - Horizontal CR, x-ray tube superior, intensifier inferior
- Ensure sterile field.
- Provide lead aprons or shields.
- Background exposure field greatest at tube end; operator should stand back away from tube region.

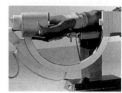

Fig. 10.11 C-arm for lateral hip. (Courtesy Philips Medical System.)

Note: Recommended setup is a reversal of this as an inferosuperior projection because of increased radiation at tube end.

Procedure Notes

_____
_____
_____
_____
_____
_____
_____
_____
_____
_____
_____
_____
_____
_____
_____
_____
_____
_____
_____
_____
_____
_____
_____
_____
_____
_____
_____
_____
_____
_____
_____
_____
_____
_____
_____
_____
_____

Appendix A: Reducing Patient Dose

There are seven common practices to reduce patient dose during radiographic procedures. They include the following:

1. **Minimize repeat radiographs:** A primary cause of repeat radiographs is poor communication between the technologist and the patient. The technologist must clearly explain the procedure to the patient. Carelessness in positioning and selection of erroneous technique factors are common causes of repeats and should be avoided. Review technical and positioning errors with other technologists and determine corrections before repeating the exposures.

2. **Correct filtration:** Filtration of the primary x-ray beam reduces exposure to the patient by preferentially absorbing low-energy "unusable" x-rays, which mainly expose the patient's skin and superficial tissue without contributing to image formation.

3. **Accurate collimation:** The practice of close collimation to only the area of interest reduces patient dose by reducing the volume of tissue directly irradiated, and the amount of accompanying scattered radiation is decreased. The technologist must not rely on positive beam limitation (PBL) collimators. They will collimate to the size of the image receptor only. Additional collimation is needed to further reduce exposure to surrounding tissues not required for the study.

4. **Shielding:** All radiosensitive tissues outside the region of interest should be shielded.

5. **Specific area shielding (gonadal and female breast shielding):** Specific area shielding is essential when radiosensitive organs, such as the thyroid gland, breasts, and gonads, are in or near the useful beam and the use of such shielding do not interfere with the objectives of the examination. The most common and most important area shielding is gonadal shielding, which significantly lowers the dose to the reproductive organs. Gonadal shields, if placed correctly, reduce the gonadal dose by 50%–90% if the gonads are in the primary x-ray field. Gonadal shielding is necessary when the region of study is within or near (2 inches [5 cm]) the primary beam.

6. **Protection of the fetus:** All women of childbearing age should be screened for the possibility of pregnancy before an x-ray examination.

320

7. **Select projections and exposure factors appropriate for the examination:** Perform projections (pending department approval) that minimize dose to radiosensitive tissues, such as the breast and eye. A PA projection will greatly reduce dose to these tissues compared with an AP projection. Select exposure factors that use highest allowable kV and lowest mAs to further reduce patient dose.

Ethical Practice in Digital Imaging: The wide dynamic range of digital imaging enables an acceptable image to be obtained with a broad range of exposure factors. During the evaluation of the quality of an image, the technologist must ensure that the exposure indicator is within the recommended range. Any attempt to process an image with a different algorithm to correct overexposure is not acceptable; it is vital that patient dose be minimized at the outset and that the ALARA (As Low As Reasonably Achievable) principle be upheld.

To maintain dose at a reasonable, consistent dose level, the following practices are recommended:

- Use protocol-specific kV ranges and mAs values for all procedures. Use as high of a kV possible.
- Monitor dose by reviewing all images.
- If the exposure indicator for a given procedure is outside of the acceptable range, review all factors, including kV, mAs, positioning, collimation, and anatomy with a supervisor or radiation safety officer (RSO).

Appendix B: Time-mA (mAs) Chart

Time in Seconds		mA (mAs in Boxes)										
		50	75	100	150	200	250	300	400	500	600	800
1/500	0.002	0.1	0.15	0.2	0.3	0.4	0.5	0.6	0.8	1.0	1.2	1.6
1/200	0.005	0.25	0.38	0.5	0.75	1.0	1.25	1.5	2.0	2.5	3.0	4.0
1/120	0.008	0.4	0.6	0.8	1.2	1.6	2.0	2.4	3.2	4.0	4.8	6.4
1/100	0.010	0.5	0.75	1.0	1.5	2.0	2.5	3.0	4.0	5.0	6.0	8.0
≈1/80	0.013	0.65	0.98	1.3	1.95	2.6	3.25	3.9	5.2	6.5	7.8	10.4
≈1/60	0.016	0.8	1.2	1.6	2.4	3.2	4.0	4.8	6.4	8.0	9.6	12.8
≈1/50	0.019	0.95	1.43	1.9	2.85	3.8	4.75	5.7	7.6	9.5	11.4	15.2
1/40	0.025	1.25	1.88	2.5	3.75	5.0	6.25	7.5	10.0	12.5	15.0	20.0
1/30	0.033	1.65	2.48	3.3	4.95	6.6	8.25	9.9	13.2	16.5	19.8	26.4
≈1/24	0.041	2.05	3.08	4.1	6.15	8.2	10.25	12.3	16.4	20.5	24.6	32.8
1/20	0.050	2.5	3.75	5.0	7.5	10.0	12.5	15.0	20.0	25.0	30.0	40.0
≈1/15	0.064	3.2	4.8	6.4	9.6	12.8	16.0	19.2	25.6	32.0	38.4	51.2
1/12	0.08	4.0	6.0	8.0	12.0	16.0	20.0	24.0	32.0	40.0	48.0	64.0
1/10	0.10	5.0	7.5	10.0	15.0	20.0	25.0	30.0	40.0	50.0	60.0	80.0
1/8	0.125	6.25	9.38	12.5	18.8	25.0	31.25	37.5	50.0	62.5	75.0	100.0
1/6	0.16	8.0	12.0	16.0	24.0	32.0	40.0	48.0	64.0	80.0	96.0	128.0
1/5	0.20	10.0	15.0	20.0	30.0	40.0	50.0	60.0	80.0	100.0	120.0	160.0
3/10	0.30	15.0	22.5	30.0	45.0	60.0	75.0	90.0	120.0	150.0	180.0	240.0
2/5	0.40	20.0	30.0	40.0	60.0	80.0	100.0	120.0	160.0	200.0	240.0	320.0
1/2	0.50	25.0	37.5	50.0	75.0	100.0	125.0	150.0	200.0	250.0	300.0	400.0
3/5	0.60	30.0	45.0	60.0	90.0	120.0	150.0	80.0	240.0	300.0	360.0	480.0
4/5	0.80	40.0	60.0	80.0	120.0	60.0	200.0	240.0	320.0	400.0	480.0	640.0

Appendix B: Time-mA (mAs) Chart

Appendix C: Exposure-Distance Conversion Chart

New SID	Original SID 36" (91 cm)	40" (102 cm)	42" (107 cm)	44" (113 cm)	48" (123 cm)	60" (153 cm)	72" (183 cm)	100" (256 cm)	120" (307 cm)
30" (76 cm)	0.7	0.6	0.5	0.5	0.4	0.3	0.2	0.1	0.1
36" (92 cm)	1.0	0.8	0.7	0.7	0.6	0.4	0.3	0.1	0.1
40" (102 cm)	1.2	1.0	0.9	0.8	0.7	0.4	0.3	0.2	0.1
42" (107 cm)	1.4	1.1	1.0	0.9	0.8	0.5	0.3	0.2	0.1
44" (113 cm)	1.5	**1.2**	1.1	1.0	0.8	0.5	0.4	0.2	0.1
46" (117 cm)	1.6	1.3	1.2	1.1	0.9	0.6	0.4	0.2	0.2
48" (123 cm)	1.8	1.4	1.3	1.2	1.0	0.6	0.4	0.2	0.2
50" (128 cm)	1.9	1.6	1.4	1.3	1.1	0.7	0.5	0.3	0.2
55" (140 cm)	2.3	1.9	1.7	1.6	1.3	0.8	0.6	0.3	0.2
60" (153 cm)	2.8	2.3	2.0	1.9	1.6	1.0	0.7	0.4	0.3
72" (183 cm)	4.0	3.2	2.9	2.7	2.3	1.4	1.0	0.5	0.4
100" (256 cm)	7.7	6.3	5.7	5.2	4.3	2.8	1.9	0.1	0.7
120" (307 cm)	11.1	9.0	8.2	7.4	6.3	4.0	2.8	1.4	1.0

Example 1: Determine mAs with SID changed from 40" to 44". (Look down the 40" column to the 44" box, and locate 1.2 as the conversion factor.)
Original mAs = 8.

Answer: 8 × 1.2 = 9.6 or 10 mAs

Example 2: A chest technique @ 72" is 6 mAs @ 90 kVp. If the SID needs to be decreased to 60", what mAs should be used if other factors remain unchanged?

Answer: Conversion factor is **0.7**. 6 mAs × .7 = 4.2 mAs

Appendix C: Exposure-Distance Conversion Chart

Appendix D: Cast Conversion Rule

A cast applied to upper or lower limbs (extremities) requires an increase in exposure. One suggested method for determining exposure compensation is to measure for the increased thickness of the part, including the cast, and adjust the exposure factors accordingly.

The above method can be used in general, but in addition to the added thickness of the cast, the different densities of cast materials also affect the required exposure adjustments. Therefore the following general cast conversion guide, which makes allowances for both the size and type of cast material, is suggested.

Increase Exposure With Cast

An upper or lower limb with a cast requires an increase in exposure. This increase depends on the thickness and type of cast, as outlined in the following table:

Cast Conversion Chart

Cast Type	Increase in Exposure*
Small-to-medium plaster	5–7 kV
Large plaster	8–10 kV
Fiberglass	3–4 kV

*To reduce patient dose, it is recommended to increase kV rather than mAs.

Example: An AP and lateral ankle were taken at 66 kV and 6 mAs demonstrating a fracture. A medium-size plaster cast was applied, and postreduction projections were ordered. What exposure factors should be used?

Answer: 73 kV @ 6 mAs (+ 7 kV)

Appendix E: Grid Ratio Conversion Chart

New Grid Ratio	Recommended kV Range	Original Grid Ratio (Original Exposure Factors)				
		Nongrid <60-70	5:1 or 6:1 60-75	8:1 70-90	12:1 70-25 (95-125)	16:1 70-125 (95-125)
Nongrid	<60-70	1	0.33	0.25	0.20 (0.17)	0.17 (0.14)
5:1 or 6:1	60-75	3	1.00	0.75	0.60	0.50
8:1	70-90	4	1.33	1.00	0.80	0.67
12:1	70-125 (95-125)	5 (6)	1.67	1.25	1.00	0.83
16:1	70-125 (95-125)	6 (7)	2.00	1.50	1.20	1.00

This conversion chart can be used for general grid conversions based on recommended mid-kV ranges of each grid type.

To use this chart, determine the correct conversion factor (multiplication number) by looking down the chart to the new grid being used, and multiply by this factor.

Example: If 7 **mAs** @ 70 kV is the technique for a shoulder using a 12:1 grid, what mAs should be used with a 5:1 portable grid?

Answer: The conversion factor for converting from 12:1 to 5:1 is **0.6.**

7 mAs × 0.6 = **4.2 mAs** @ 70 kV

To check your answer, convert the other way from a 5:1 to a 12:1 grid. An increase in technique would be needed, and the conversion factor is **1.67.** (4.2 mAs × 1.67 = **7 mAs**, the original technique for the 12:1 grid.)

Appendix F: Initials (Abbreviations), Technical Terms, and Acronyms

The following are the more common initials (abbreviations) and acronyms used in imaging departments today and as used in this pocket handbook and in the 9th edition Bontrager Textbook.

General Positioning/Anatomy Terms

AC joints	Acromioclavicular joints
AP, PA	Anteroposterior, posteroanterior projections
ASIS	Anterior superior iliac spine (pelvis landmark)
DP, PD	Dorsoplantar and plantodorsal
LAO, RAO	Left and right anterior oblique projections
LPO, RPO	Left and right posterior oblique projections
MCP	Midcoronal plane (plane dividing the body into anterior and posterior halves)
MSP	Midsagittal plane (plane dividing the body into right and left halves)
SC joints	Sternoclavicular joints
SI joints	Sacroiliac joints
SMV, VSM	Submentovertex or verticosubmental projections

Abdominal Procedure Terms

BE	Barium enema
CNS	Central nervous system
CSF	Cerebrospinal fluid
CTC	Computed tomography colonoscopy
ERCP	Endoscopic retrograde cholangiopancreatography
GB	Gallbladder
GI, UGI, LGI	Gastrointestinal, upper and lower GI
IVP	Intravenous pyelogram (older term)
IVU	Intravenous urogram (accurate term)
KUB	Kidneys, ureters, bladder (abdomen projection)
NPO	Nil per os (nothing by mouth)
PTC	Percutaneous transhepatic cholangiography
RLQ, LLQ	Right and left lower quadrant
RUQ, LUQ	Right and left upper quadrant
SBS	Small bowel series
VC	Virtual colonoscopy

Technical Terms

AEC	Automatic exposure controls
Analog	Film-screen imaging system
CR	Central ray (for positioning centering)
CR	Computed radiography—using image plates (IP)
CT	Computed tomography
DF	Digital fluoroscopy
DR	Digital radiography (cassetteless)
FS	Focal spot (large or small)
HIS	Hospital information system
IP	Image plates (used with CR)
IR	Image receptor (film/screen or digital)
Landscape	Crosswise (IR orientation to patient)
MRI	Magnetic resonance imaging
OID	Object image receptor distance
PACS	Picture archiving and communications system
PBL	Positive beam limitation (collimation)
PET	Positron emission tomography
PSP	Photostimulable phosphor plate receptor (either cassette or cassetteless)
Portrait	Lengthwise (IR orientation to patient)
RIS	Radiology information system
SID	Source image-receptor distance
TT	Tabletop (non-bucky)

Terms Related to Joints of Limbs (Extremities)

ACL, PCL	Anterior and posterior cruciate ligaments (knee)
CMC	Carpometacarpal (wrist)
DIP	Distal interphalangeal (hand or foot)
IP	Interphalangeal (hand or foot)
LCL, MCL	Lateral and medial collateral ligaments (knee)
MCP	Metacarpophalangeal (hand)
MTP	Metatarsophalangeal (foot)
PIP	Proximal interphalangeal (hand or foot)
TMT	Tarsometatarsal (foot)

Terms Related to Cranium and Facial Bones

AML	Acanthiomeatal line
EAM	External acoustic meatus

GAL	Glabelloalveolar line
GML	Glabellomeatal line
IOML	Infraorbital-meatal line
IPL	Interpupillary line
LML	Lips-meatal line (modified Waters projection)
MML	Mentomeatal line (Waters projection)
OML	Orbitomeatal line
SOG	Supraorbital groove
TEA	Top of ear attachment
TMJ	Temporomandibular joints